Testimonials

"This easy to read, sensible and insightful book, offers practical information and advice simply and compassionately given for all stages of the condition. This will be a great resource which can be picked up in times of need and can be used to jot down questions, ideas and useful strategies along the journey that can be helpful reminders when talking with healthcare professionals. Knowing that you are not alone on this journey and that there are people out there like Jane with the expertise, knowledge, empathy and the passion to offer this support means a great deal. Jane lets us know that none of us are experts, but with kindness and wisdom helps us to do our best and advises that we all need to be kind to ourselves and ask for help when we need it."

—**Carol Maddock, Daughter**

"Jane's compassion and warmth shines through her words. I believe that it will be a comfort to families/ caregivers who are experiencing the fear of a diagnosis and will offer an anchor when they're unsure of how to communicate. I think it will also be a helpful tool for professionals to help them educate extended family and friends to help them understand what's happening and manage expectations. Jane has a real knack for taking the 'edge' off a difficult subject through her reassuring tone and practical tips. This gives people a pathway to follow through the 'mist' as you would say- a guiding light"

—**Mari Evans Mental Health Nurse Consultant.**

"Finding the Light In Dementia has been invaluable and has helped us know what to do and how. We are currently caring for my 90-year-old Mum together in her home and with all the challenges that later Stage Alzheimer's bring, this book has been a great source of wisdom on how to tailor our approach. We have used the book to provide a consistent approach to her care. All professional home caregivers would also benefit from reading this to enable them to provide the best care possible in their role. It's also a book that reminds us to look after ourselves!"

—Angharad and Anthony Brown,
Daughter and Son-in-Law, Family Caregivers

"This little book is a life saver for people who have dementia and their caregivers, families and friends. I think it should be given out by every professional who gives the initial diagnosis. People need something to grasp, and the sensitivity, simplicity and emotion contained in this book may help them cope better."

— Lorraine Morgan, Nurse Consultant

"It's absolutely amazing, I think it should be compulsory reading for everybody at the start of dementia. I wish it had been around when my husband started developing it"

—Elizabeth Cox, Wife and Caregiver

"This is an insightfully wonderful book for both caregivers and professionals alike. 'Finding The Light In Dementia' helps to calm the overwhelming feelings that come with a diagnosis of Dementia or Alzheimer's. It is almost as if Jane has gently taken your hand in hers and is walking alongside you, encouraging you through this new chapter of your life. She has provided wonderful information; plus note pages at the end of the chapters for you to keep a record of the questions you want to ask the Doctor. This book is a much needed gift to yourself."

—Carole Fawcett, MPCC, Counsellor

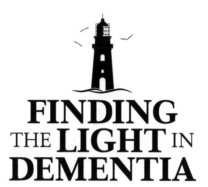

FINDING
THE **LIGHT** IN
DEMENTIA

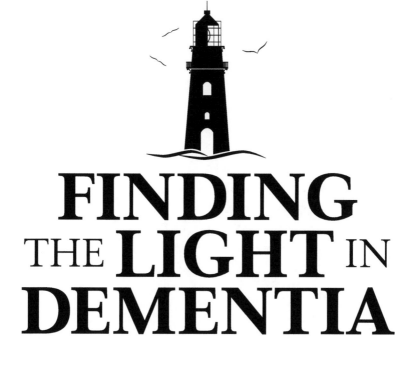

FINDING THE LIGHT IN DEMENTIA

A Guide for Families, Friends and Caregivers

JANE M. MULLINS

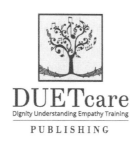

DUETcare
Dignity Understanding Empathy Training

PUBLISHING

The information in this book should not be treated as a substitute for professional medical and/or legal advice. Use of this book is at the reader's discretion. Neither the author nor publisher can be held responsible for any damage, loss or claim arising out of the use or misuse, of the suggestions made.

The names and identifying details of the individuals in the case studies have been changed to respect their anonymity.

Visit my website www.findingthelightindementia.com

Publisher's Cataloging-in-Publication Data
Names: Mullins, Jane M., author.
Title: Finding the light in dementia: a guide for families, friends, and caregivers / Jane M. Mullins.
Description: Includes bibliographical references | Cardiff, UK: DUETcare Publishing, 2017.
Identifiers: ISBN 978-1-9999268-0-9
Subjects: LCSH Dementia--Patients--Care. | Alzheimer's disease--Patients--Care. | Caregivers--psychology. | Patient Care--ethics. | Social Support. | BISAC HEALTH & FITNESS / Diseases / Alzheimer's & Dementia | FAMILY & RELATIONSHIPS / Life Stages / Later Years
Classification: LCC RC523 .M85 2017 | DDC 362.1/96831--dc23

Edited by Carole Fawcett www.amindfulconnection.com
Book Design by AuthorSupport.com

Dedicated to:

Elizabeth and Roger
Beti and David
Gillian and Denys

Be a lamp, or a lifeboat, or a ladder.
Help someone's soul heal.

RUMI

Contents

Author's Note

Receiving a diagnosis of dementia comes with a multitude of emotions: fear, devastation, shock, panic, resentment and bemusement. All of these feelings are caused by uncertainty about what lies ahead and having to face up to an unknown future.

Finding the Light is here to offer hope and comfort by helping you to understand what is happening to your loved one living with dementia. Once you can understand why their behaviour may change, this book guides you with practical, creative tips to see through the mist of dementia and helps you re-connect with them and yourself. *Finding the Light* suggests taking small steps to adopt enjoyable approaches to help overcome some of the difficulties you may be experiencing.

I will explain about how dementia may affect your loved one in relation to space and time, sensory changes, communication difficulties and differences in thinking and reasoning. *Finding the Light* goes on to explore how you can communicate and re-connect with them by making subtle changes in the environment, whether indoors or outdoors, being aware of your body language and creating sensory life stories that make the most of the senses.

Following the simple activities and tips recommended here may help to keep your relationships vibrant and healthy. They may also help toward slowing down your partner's* deterioration. By understanding what happens when somebody has dementia, you will learn to be more empathic and re-develop a connection with your partner and with yourself, thereby helping to maintain love and dignity. *Finding the Light* also helps you to recognise your needs and offers steps to self-care. By caring for yourself, you are in a better place to care for others.

This book is not meant to replace your doctor. Dementia affects people individually and different stages will come with different issues; therefore, the advice here is general and does not necessarily suggest that your partner will experience all of the changes discussed.

---

* I will refer to your loved one as partner in the sense of care partner throughout the book

Introduction

Dementia is a term for a number of symptoms that affect the brain due to disease or the presence of small strokes. It is progressive in nature which means that the individual affected will experience ongoing deterioration of their condition. There are a number of different types of dementia that include Alzheimer's disease; vascular dementia; Lewy body dementia; frontotemporal dementia and Parkinson's disease dementia as well as rarer conditions. The person diagnosed will experience different symptoms that depend on the type of dementia and where the damage in the brain occurs. For the purpose of this book, I have covered the most common effects that can occur in all types of dementia and may affect people at different times. Your partner may not experience all the symptoms noted in this book, but it is important to understand what is happening to them and how you can help at all stages of their condition.

Having a diagnosis of dementia can be a frightening experience often leading to feelings of anxiety and uncertainty for the future. Chapter one in *Finding the Light* offers guidance and practical advice about what positive plans you need to make together.

People who have dementia may become disoriented to time and space. They need to be in a relaxing and familiar environment surrounded by people who know them or know their lifestory in order to feel safe and secure. They also need to be around people who understand the nature of dementia. Involve their friends and family; children can be particularly intuitive and offer a blanket of hope and a great source of love. Language is often affected by dementia, so *Finding the Light* introduces ways we can communicate beyond speaking. Chapter Two will help you make the most of non-verbal forms of communication and find ways of understanding each other. This includes using your senses and body language and learning to find your connection at a deeper spiritual level.

Memory and awareness of time and place can be affected by dementia. This can include forgetting, repetitive behaviour, failing to recognise people, not understanding time and getting lost. *Finding the Light* helps you to understand what your partner is experiencing. Chapter Three provides suggestions to overcome these difficulties and Chapter Four offers ways to stimulate memories together to help you both find joy in shared remembering.

Judgement may be impaired by dementia: this can include not being able to recognise risks, such as knowing that a hot cup of tea may scald, or how to dress appropriately for the weather. Dementia can also affect how and what a person is able to see in the world around them. *Finding the Light* explains how, with your understanding, you can gently guide your partner in the decisions they make while helping you understand what they may be experiencing. Chapter Five will introduce you to some ideas to help your partner feel safe, secure and content while maintaining their independence for as long as possible.

Eating, drinking and sleeping can be affected by dementia. *Finding the Light* shows how good nutrition, hydration and sleep can help you both keep well and maintain some balance in your lives together. Chapters Six and Seven offer some tips and advice to help you both stay rested and nourished.

Appearance and a sense of who we are can change due to dementia. *Finding the Light* identifies the difficulties that can occur when attending to appearance and personal care. Chapter Eight helps provide practical suggestions to help your partner keep their dignity and sense of self-worth.

Changes in behaviour can occur when living with dementia. *Finding the Light* explains mood changes and fixed beliefs, which can be due to fear and frustration as well as changes in the brain. Chapters Nine and Ten explain what might be happening to your partner. These chapters offer approaches to help minimise the difficulties they experience and to see that there may be a message behind this behaviour that needs to be responded to sensitively.

When caring for someone living with dementia, we

tend to forget about our own needs, and this can lead to emotional, physical and social problems for ourselves. We may become resentful, experience emotions that make us feel guilty, have our own health problems and become isolated from our friends. Chapter Eleven suggests positive steps to self-care while caring for your partner.

There may come a time when you will need to consider professional help in caring for your partner. Chapter Twelve offers advice about befriending, care in the home and what to consider when looking at a care home, either for respite or on a long-term basis. This also includes advice in the event of a hospital admission. It gently helps you to see the benefits of asking for help and shows how you can continue to connect together and both stay well when other caregivers are involved.

The nature of dementia means that your partner's condition waxes and wanes as time goes on. This book helps you to think about being creative and flexible in your caring and recommends that you consider the suggestions here. If you have found that some strategies no longer work, it doesn't mean that they won't work in the future.......keep an open mind. You might want to consider a trial and error approach to solving any of the difficulties you both experience.

The ethos of this book is to help you connect with and care for your partner and for yourself. Include your family and friends and ask them to read *Finding the Light* too, so that they can feel confident and become more involved. Whether you're a spouse, partner, daughter, son, sibling, parent or friend, this book is for you.

I know how busy you are, so for quick reference, the main points to remember are summarised at the end of each chapter, alongside some notes pages for you to write key points about what works for both of you, e.g. noting your partner's likes and dislikes (I would recommend putting a date alongside these notes as preferences may change over time). It can also act as an essential guide for any other caregiver or family member who spends time with your partner.

I have provided a question sheet at the back of the book that gives you space to write down any questions you need to ask your doctor, health care professional and/or legal representative. There is also room for you to jot down their responses, as we can be overwhelmed at clinic appointments and forget all that they have told us. Keeping this information in one place will help reduce your stress. Just make sure that you take this book along with you to every appointment. You could always ask the professionals to write down their advice for you on these pages.

CHAPTER ONE

A Diagnosis of Dementia, What Now?

How to face up to the situation and make positive plans for the future

Even though the darkest phase be it thick or thin, always someone marches brave here beneath my skin.

K.D. LANG

If your partner has just received a diagnosis of dementia you are probably both feeling scared and uncertain about what lies ahead. If you have children living at home there will be an added concern about how you and your partner's roles as parents will change. Be kind to yourselves, as you will need a little time to get used to this. It is usually helpful to talk to family and friends openly and ask for their support. Be mindful that these need to be positive people who have a good relationship with you both.

"I just remember sitting down in the hospital and being called in by the nurse, Joe was fidgeting, he was very nervous. The doctor was lovely and made us feel comfortable and then all I heard was the word dementia......I don't remember anything else, she was talking but my head was swimming, her voice echoed through me. Joe helped me into the car and as he drove, my mind went into overdrive...what about the kids? Will I still be able to work? How will I keep everything going in the house? Will my friends come and see me? Everything was a blur and panic set in. I just cried and cried for what seemed like days. But slowly with the help of my nurse and my family I started to feel a bit better and now I take it a day at a time. I find it really helps to talk."

– **Rachel**

Once you have had some time to get used to the diagnosis it is important to take some control and start to make plans together. There is currently no cure for dementia, but much can be done to help you and your partner live a meaningful life and remain well. *Finding the Light* is here to explain what can be happening to your partner and answer many questions to help you both along the way. It is important that you help them remain as independent as possible and encourage them to continue to do tasks and be involved in everyday life. By keeping them stimulated and active, you will remind them that they still have a great purpose, which will help them feel valued. By motivating your partner to stay occupied you may actually help towards slowing down their deterioration. Focus on what your partner can do and not what they cannot do. It is very important to listen to them and to allow them and yourself to voice concerns. Do not brush it under the carpet, it is by talking through feelings and facing up to the diagnosis that positive plans can be put in place.

Firstly, speak with your doctor about addressing any support and possible treatment and care needs. Some medications are licensed for certain types of dementia that may help to temporarily slow down the disease and thereby manage the symptoms. Whether your partner will be offered these will depend on their medical history. Where diagnosed with vascular dementia, speak to your doctor about minimising the risk of possible further strokes such as reducing high blood pressure, adopting a healthy Mediterranean diet and taking part in gentle exercise. There is much that can be achieved through living healthily with fresh air, exercise and good nutrition.

It is quite likely that you will both be feeling anxious, I would certainly recommend trying to get outdoors together and go on walks to help your moods and to help you both get into the habit of making healthy decisions, (there is much research to support this and you will note that I suggest this in a number of the chapters throughout this book). It may also be worth finding out about psychological therapies such as cognitive behavioural therapy (CBT)* to help with low mood and anxiety that may occur due to the dementia. Your doctor may be able to recommend a psychotherapist or a counsellor to help you both. *Finding the Light* will also prove invaluable by introducing ways to keep your partner mentally and physically stimulated and may even help slow down the progression of their dementia.

It is important to work together to plan for the future. Planning ahead may help to avoid difficult situations arising and sometimes even avert a crisis in terms of care, welfare and finances. You will both need to explore your options with regard to putting affairs in order since your partner's ability to make decisions will be affected over time. Make sure when discussing such legal and financial matters, that your partner feels safe and that their feelings are listened to, with no confrontation involved.

I would recommend sitting together more than once to discuss your partner's choices and decisions in relation to finances and future care with them. This may not always be easy but if you can both make such plans it will help you in the future. Maybe start off with writing down what they want and what they don't want. For example, they may have specific religious and/or cultural beliefs that may influence what they eat or how they worship or

---

* http://www.nhs.uk/Conditions/Cognitive-behavioural-therapy/Pages/Introduction.aspx
https://www.ncbi.nlm.nih.gov/pubmedhealth/PMH0072481/
https://www.healthdirect.gov.au/cognitive-behaviour-therapy-cbt
https://adaa.org/finding-help/treatment/therapy

they may wish to avoid certain medical treatment. It is important that their choices are documented and while decisions may change, you will both have taken some control in future planning.

I have found that many people have experienced financial difficulties due to internet banking and shopping and have been inundated with credit card applications and people trying to sell products over the phone and online. People who have dementia are vulnerable and often exploited. I would recommend blocking your phone number and email address to outside sources (look up on the internet and type in "how to block your phone number and email address") and just keep your access available to trusted family and friends.

You should speak to a legal advisor to help with planning your financial and welfare future such as gaining advice about power of attorney and avoiding getting into debt or being the victim of scamming, (where people fraudulently extort money). It is also worth speaking to them about living wills and advance care planning to make sure that your partner's wishes are respected. If you don't have an existing advisor, contact your local dementia charity, they should be able to support you in your decisions and direct you to the help you need.

We live in a world of having to use remote controls, computers and mobile phones that require remembering multiple passwords, numbers and codes. Whether it is supermarket shopping, banking or accessing media we are becoming more reliant on technology. This can cause much confusion and stress when we struggle to remember such numbers. Recent research has shown that with the right support and use of memory strategies some people who have dementia are still able to find ways to use these devices and recall such information (see chapter three). But you will need to consider keeping these passwords/numbers/codes in a safe place in the event of forgetting them.

Try and limit your workload by setting up direct debits with your utility companies to automatically pay your bills and if you do have any other financial transactions write them on a separate calendar or diary for marking when payments are due and when they have been paid. You will feel less overwhelmed if you are organised and have a day-to-day routine. You may find that a large diary can help where all correspondence can be kept in one place and dealt with. Get in the habit of crossing off tasks that have been completed. Keep all your important documents in one place, maybe a small filing cabinet or box. If your partner still wants to be involved with the paperwork it may be an idea to make photocopies.

If your partner is still working, you will need to consider discussing the diagnosis with their human resources/personnel department and occupational health. Depending on their job and how their dementia is affecting them, they should be able to offer some flexible working conditions or plans to help support your partner. They may also help with reviewing pensions and possible future options. A diagnosis of dementia does not necessarily mean that they have to give up their job immediately but the roles that they undertake may change over time. If you work, I would recommend that you also speak to your employer as you may need time away for hospital appointments and/or as a support for your partner.

You and your partner will also need to speak to your doctor about whether they can continue to drive at the present moment. A diagnosis of dementia does not mean that your partner's driving licence will be automatically taken from them but it is important to know that at some point their condition will affect their driving ability. This is always a difficult subject to broach. In most countries the law requires drivers or their doctors to report their diagnosis to the appropriate vehicle licensing and motorists' associations". I would recommend that you and your partner have regular honest conversations with your doctor about discussing the risks and benefits of driving and start to consider alternative methods of transport. It is important that your partner is able to express their feelings and may be worth asking your doctor to refer you both for ongoing emotional support.

If you have a young family you are undoubtedly going to be concerned about how the diagnosis will impact on

" https://www.dementia.org.au/files/NSW-Staying-on-th-move-with-dementia-booklet.pdf
https://www.alz.org/national/documents/statements_driving.pdf
https://www.alzheimers.org.uk/download/downloads/id/729/living_with_dementia_-_driving.pdf

them. While the news is distressing, children and teens may actually be relieved to know that their loved one's behaviour is caused by a disease and that <u>they</u> are not the cause. It is better to be open and honest with them so they can continue to feel trust toward you and they may learn how to manage their emotions more effectively when the family pulls together. Make sure that you explain to them about the diagnosis in a calm way and give some simple examples of how the dementia may affect your partner, such as forgetting names and losing words. Remember it is important to remind them of all that your partner is still able to do so that you do not all focus too much on their difficulties.

Give your children plenty of hugs and reassurance, involve them and give them the opportunity to ask questions at all times and to express their feelings[***]. Encourage them to read *Finding the Light*. Suggest positive ways to come together include creating family life stories (see chapter four) and getting involved in current activities, walks together and hobbies. This will help you all stay connected to your partner/parent and give you some practical solutions for the present and the future.

It is important that you do not face this alone, encourage your friends and family to visit and be involved. Over time you may need to look for some additional support such as from a befriender, who are volunteers that come

---

[***] https://www.allyballybee.org/category/dementia-videos/
http://www.alz.org/living_with_alzheimers_just_for_kids_and_teens.asp

to help as friendly visitors into your home. By involving more people who know you and your partner well and understand the nature of dementia (by reading this book) you can continue to live well together.

I hope that this chapter will help you towards coming to terms with the diagnosis of dementia by offering helpful guidance and support in what to do next. You will see that *Finding the Light* provides a positive outlook and will give you more confidence to care and support your partner by explaining what may be happening to them and how they may feel. When referring to the chapters in this book you will learn invaluable strategies for the coming years. Be aware that your partner may not experience all that is covered in this book, however the information is here, should the need arise, with a view to helping you both stay connected.

Summary of Chapter One

Main Points to remember about planning for the future

- Take time to listen to each other and focus on making positive plans.
- Involve family & friends, it is much better to face this together than brush it all under the carpet. Keep socialising as this can help to keep you both well.
- Plan to follow a healthy lifestyle i.e. make a point of having a daily walk in the fresh air and follow a Mediterranean diet, i.e. plenty of fresh fruit, vegetables and fish.
- Focus on your partner's strengths and not what they cannot do.
- Find out what your partner wants.
- Speak to your doctor about any possible treatments available and gain advice about driving, work and care needs (where applicable). Ask them to refer you both for counselling and support.
- Consult a trusted legal representative to discuss financial and welfare issues and make plans.
- Speak with your partner's work and occupational health department.

- Organise ways of remembering passwords, numbers and codes.
- Block unknown callers to emails and phones, only allowing access from trusted family and friends.
- Read through *Finding the Light* for plenty of suggestions. Key things to remember are to keep in touch with family and friends, eat well, gentle daily exercise and keep occupied with meaningful activities.
- Use the next few pages to make any notes relevant to you both.
- Use the question sheets at the back of this book for consultations with your partner's doctor and legal representative.

Use the notes pages to make any personal comments from your discussions with your partner, family & friends. You may find that writing a diary may also help.

NOTES

Date: **Comment:**

NOTES

Date: Comment:

NOTES

Date: **Comment:**

CHAPTER TWO

Communicating from the Heart

How to find ways to help you communicate well together

My heart speaks and yet my tongue is mute.

RUMI

At some stage, people who have dementia may experience problems with communication. This can be in the form of being able to communicate their wishes (expressive) and/or being able to understand what somebody is saying to them (receptive). This can be intermittent or constant and can be extremely frustrating and frightening at times. Often people know what they want to say but cannot find the right words. Many times, I have heard them say that the word is on "the tip of my tongue".

"You see what it's doing to me now? I've got to wait until I can... not wait, but I've got to keep trying....... I can see it and then it'll come.... I can see the place now, I'm trying to find the name, that......no I should say it as I remember it, rather than try to get it more perfect.........damn...this thing stops me speaking."

– Michael

Also, the brain may affect the speed at which thoughts and words are processed, and this has an effect on both understanding and conveying messages. Being stressed can make this much worse, so it is important to give your partner time to express themselves and not rush them or finish their sentences for them. When we slow down, we can take more notice of non-verbal communication: this includes facial expressions, gestures, posture and movement. If your partner is sitting, sit at their level and keep eye contact, call them gently by their name, wait patiently for them to respond. We have to learn to sit in silence sometimes and realise that we can communicate without words. Direct questioning may make them feel under pressure. Try a different approach. As an example, you may wish to say to them "the toilet is here" instead of "do you need the toilet?".

Be aware of possible hearing loss and don't shout or over-exaggerate, making sure background noise is at a minimum. You can speak a little slower but make sure that the natural rhythm of your speech is maintained.

Also make sure that if your partner wears a hearing aid, it is in working order and you have contact with your audiology clinic. Ask for help from family and friends with hospital and clinic visits.

I have found that often where speech and language deteriorate, the language of emotions steps in.

"I have to accept that my voice is a part of me and that's it; it's my voice. If anyone is thinking of me, the voice is still here, just about (tearful)."

– George

It is important to recognise your partner's need to communicate and here you will need to adopt more creative ways to understand one another. If you have been together for a long time, you probably communicate on a deeper level without realising. If a person appears distressed, they may not be able to express that they are hungry, in pain or need to use the toilet. Feelings are often communicated more easily than facts and people who have dementia may speak more in metaphor or skirt around those lost words by using other well-used phrases. It is important to listen to what is being communicated, not solely concentrating on the words being spoken, but more on the feelings being conveyed. Validating feelings is so important, such as "I know it must be hard not being able to tell me what you want to say, but I am listening to you". Your partner should also respond well if you mirror their body language and the rhythm, intonation and speed of their speech. By mirroring them you are effectively saying to them that you are like them. This helps retain trust and helps you to connect together. They may then be able to mirror you in return.

It is worth noting that when you take on the body language associated with an emotion, you will start to feel the emotion. So even though you may be feeling tired and your mood may be low, try and *be* together with your partner and sit as upright in your chair as physically possible, roll your shoulders back and turn your face into a smile. You may find that your partner may do the same. I have known people break into laughter in the midst of difficult times just by altering their body language. Slapstick films show the power of non-verbal communication in making us laugh and in fact, clowning and playfulness has been shown to reduce stress and provide laughter and joy to those who struggle to communicate[*].

Also, be aware that whatever your partner is saying, their reality is real to them. Try to avoid contradicting or correcting them. If they insist on going out in the rain without a coat, their reality may be very different to yours. Try to say to them "I believe it is raining outside" – that way, you are being honest but not challenging or contradicting them. While I don't wish this book to become a list of do's and don'ts, there are some things that we can end up doing naturally that may not help the

---

[*] https://www.agingcare.com/articles/laughter-and-humor-with-caregiving-148553.htm

situation and may contribute to the dementia. It is therefore, worth trying the approaches recommended here. I have often heard people speaking about the person in front of them, as if they are not there. Many times, care partners have been known to say words such as "he's gone", "he's just here in body" or "she doesn't know who I am, I've lost her". This is often felt because it may be harder to communicate and get a response that we understand from them. Talking about someone in front of them without including them can contribute to the dementia as it may make them feel invisible and worthless. The person is still there, although it is so hard to come to terms with not being able to communicate with them in ways that we always have. We, therefore, need to take a new approach.

"I found that my mother was going out with the tide, and so I followed her into the sea."

– Martha

Avoid talking about your partner in front of them as if they are not there. You may know them better than anyone else, but they still exist inside and still have feelings, despite their inability to express them. People can also withdraw and become more apathetic and depressed if they are being ignored or talked about.

"I'd like to be thought of as a person and not as somebody as dementia. What I am trying to say is that I am still me, it doesn't matter whether I can no longer remember exactly who I am...what I am doing underneath I am still me...... mmm because people look at you, and they think well... you're going to be different, at least I don't think I am.... I am probably a bit more irritable (tearful)."

– Anne

Unless your partner actively wants to practice, try to avoid testing your partner's memory, this can highlight their difficulties and can make them feel a multitude of emotions, from anxiety to distress, frustration to depression. They may or may not be able show these feelings to you. Don't forget that your partner is still there, the person is still present. We have to think about walking in their shoes and imagine how we would feel.

When people come to visit, you may need to help your partner by prompting them. For instance, instead of asking them if they remember their granddaughter's name, say something like: "Hello love, your granddaughter Jessica has come to see you". That way, you are prompting them about the name of the person and their relationship to them. They may very well remember their face and that the person represents someone meaningful to them. We have to move away from worrying about the facts and move towards love, feeling and being in the moment. If your family members live far away and you don't get the opportunity to see them often, it might be a good idea to get them to make tape recordings of their voices, a good idea is to ask them to tell stories of their past experiences. Keep a photograph of them at hand when listening to them, this can be an enjoyable pastime for both you and your partner. You may also find that where your partner's 'mother tongue' is different to what was spoken as an adult, they may revert back to their original language.

There may come a time when you find that your partner has difficulty in answering open questions such as "do you want a cup of tea?". They may say "yes" but actually mean "no" and vice versa. Try saying to them "let's have a cup of tea". By doing so, you include them in your plans but don't put them under pressure to answer. You will soon know by their body language whether they actually want the drink.

If your partner repeats themselves frequently, firstly you need to see if you can help them and understand their needs, as it often means that something is on their mind that hasn't been resolved. They may be thirsty, hungry, need the toilet or be in pain. You may want to say to them something like, "I think I'll have a drink of water, why don't you have one?" or "I think I'll go to the toilet, why don't you go first?". Repetitive speech and behaviour can often occur and you will find strategies throughout the book to help you understand the reasons why and how you can help reduce the stress caused by it.

There is no doubt that there will be times when you feel frustrated and tired but try to respond gently to your partner. There is a big difference between reacting and responding. We can often react immediately and without thinking, which can lead to negative feelings. Whereas when we respond, we take a moment to think things through and are less likely to show frustration. Be present with them, face them on the same level and maintain eye contact. Take a moment to be still and mindful, and try to learn to respond with love, answering the question being asked. The use of picture cards may be helpful here. If they are unable to say what they need, they may be able to point to a picture that depicts their message. Be careful that they don't feel patronised when doing this. It may or may not work depending on whether they are able to see or recognise the picture.

Include your partner in conversations by speaking with them directly, face them and make eye contact. Make sure that other people learn to do the same and discourage them if they talk over your partner's head or speak about them as if they are not present. You will find that you have learned ways that can help your connection and show others the best way to communicate at the same time.

and BREATHE..........

Communication is so much more than words: being in the moment can help to maintain your connection to each other.

Take time to do this and forget about the chores for the moment. By breathing mindfully together, you are communicating on a much deeper level, which can help to reduce your stress. This helps you to keep that meaningful connection between the two of you.

If you find yourself feeling stressed, try this quick exercise below:

> • Try to sit quietly together and listen to your partner's breathing, listen to your breathing and try to mirror theirs, then slow your breathing down.
> • As you breathe in, count to three, and as you breathe out, count to three. Keep doing this for a few minutes.
> • You may find that their breathing slows too.

Don't always feel that you have to speak all the time. While it's important to maintain verbal communication and for your partner to hear words and word sounds, non-verbal cues such as gestures, facial expressions and body language can convey a message more effectively. Music is a wonderful way of helping us communicate.

"Music can lift us out of depression or move us to tears—it is a remedy, a tonic, orange juice for the ear. But for many of my neurological patients, music is even more—it can provide access, even when no medication can, to movement, to speech, to life. For them, music is not a luxury, but a necessity."

– Dr. Oliver Sacks

Put a favourite song on and let the vibration do the work. I'm sure feet will start tapping and some movement will happen. There is much research that shows the positive effect of music for those who have dementia. Ask your family and friends to help you create a playlist of your partner's favourite songs, they may enjoy listening to them through headphones. In the meantime, ask them to create one for you too.

"I came home one day and couldn't believe my eyes. Sheila had not spoken for the past two years and was now singing along to some golden oldies her new carer had put on our record player; she was copying her, doing the actions. Her eyes lit up and she seemed to come alive. At first, I felt bad because I didn't think to do this myself. I have been too tired to think beyond helping her wash, dress and eat in the day, but now I realise there is still life in us both. I try to keep the music going whenever I can: it helps us both together and helps when I need to care for her and makes me feel good."

– John

Where possible, keep socialising: involve family and friends. Check your local paper or internet for local memory clubs and cafés. There has recently been a rise in singing groups which can be very uplifting for all involved.

I hope that this chapter has explained how your

partner's ability to communicate can change and how that can make them feel. I have also shown you that by staying calm, taking time and using non-verbal communication you may help you both stay connected. The following pages summarise the main points and give you the opportunity to write down what works for you and your partner.

SUMMARY OF CHAPTER TWO

How dementia affects communication

- Difficulty finding words and expressing oneself
- Difficulty understanding what is being said
- The brain becomes slower at processing, so everything takes longer to understand or to say
- People often withdraw due to embarrassment, when people are impatient or when it is too much effort
- Often friends and family don't know how to communicate and visit less frequently

Approaches to help communication

- Take time
- Be in the moment

- Practice breathing together
- Maintain eye contact on the same level
- Listen to emotions being conveyed
- Clarify feelings
- Mirror body language and breathing
- Avoid contradicting
- Picture cards may help
- Use sight, hearing, taste, smell, touch and movement to help with your communication
- Do not speak over your partner's head or ignore them
- Use humour and mime
- Let others see how you communicate and encourage them to do the same

NOTES

Date: Comment:

_____   _____

_____   _____

_____   _____

_____   _____

_____   _____

_____   _____

_____   _____

_____   _____

_____   _____

_____   _____

_____   _____

_____   _____

_____   _____

_____   _____

_____   _____

_____   _____

_____   _____

_____   _____

_____   _____

_____   _____

*Use these pages to make any personal notes about
ways that help you both communicate.*

NOTES

Date:	Comment:

NOTES

Date: Comment:

NOTES

Date:	Comment:

NOTES

Artist/composer	Name of song/music

*Write down a list of music together that your partner
may like and ask your family/friends to help you record
them as a playlist to listen to with headphones.*

NOTES

Artist/composer	Name of song/music

NOTES

Artist/composer	Name of song/music

Write down a playlist for yourself.

NOTES

Artist/composer	Name of song/music

CHAPTER THREE

Using Memories to Keep in Touch

Creative approaches to stimulate memory and help with day to day living

Sometimes you may never know the value of a moment until it becomes a memory.

DR SEUSS

This chapter will explain a little about memory and how it can be affected by dementia. The person living with dementia may be able to remember their own history and retain their memory for events and life experiences, but it is often short-term memory (STM) that can be involved first. STM is responsible for temporarily storing information in the brain to allow us to perform tasks when remembering a sequence of actions. This includes understanding what is going on in the present; being able to reason and learn new things; plus being able to complete tasks. That is why a person who has dementia may repeat themselves within a very short space of time, forget what they were doing or saying and struggle with everyday chores and jobs. STM can be as short as 12 seconds.

Try and imagine how many stages there are to making a cup of tea, if you forget one part of the sequence, such as not turning the kettle on, the whole action is affected and the tea is ruined. As you can imagine, this can be very frustrating for the person experiencing short term memory loss and the more stressed they feel, the harder it is to recall or remember the information required to complete a task. Your patience and understanding will allow the person to work through the 'mist' of the moment. If your partner is getting upset, comfort them and think about creative ways of communicating with them in order to understand what they are attempting to say or do. Try and guide them in completing the task without fully taking over, they may just need a little prompting.

Help them relax with gentle touch and eye contact by being on their level, showing them, you are interested. If you are asking them to do something, break the task into small chunks encouraging them to concentrate on one thing at a time; giving short instructions and repeating by demonstrating the task. By following this approach, you are helping them to continue undertaking such tasks which will impact on their feelings of being useful and having a purpose.

Memory can also be affected in other ways, such as forgetting the names of places and recognising people and objects. Many times, people have described their dementia to me as a feeling of wading through "cotton wool" when trying to think and remember.

"Though memories are good, it was my life that was me. I was at home, I never had anyone and to find all of a sudden it takes away what you feel and can do, but it cuts your enjoyment and it cuts the fact that you feel that you are no longer you and not in control of what you can do or can say – I want to bang my head and get rid of the noise, it's all so fuzzy."

– Harry

If a friend approaches your partner and it is clear that they are struggling to recognise them or remember their name, try saying, "Hello Jim, you and (your partner's name) had such a great time working together in the office at (name of place of work)". By doing this you have saved your partner from feeling embarrassed, given them time to process the information and prompted them. This will give them some breathing space to go on and continue the conversation.

People who have dementia are often unable to visualise people and places during conversations. Many times,

I have heard caregivers say to me that they had a difficult time getting their partner to come to the memory clinic. By the time they eventually arrived they would be shattered while their partner would be charming and happy to see us (as we often gave them the VIP treatment, enjoying a cup of tea and biscuits in our waiting room; decked out with armchairs and memorabilia). This was usually because when their care partner was trying to get them ready to leave home they were unable to remember who we were or what we looked like until they saw us again, (Just think, that when we are going to a place, we can envisage the scene, the journey to get there and the people involved. People who have dementia may lose this ability.)

I was talking to a woman at the local Forget Me Not Group. She and her husband arrived late and she was very harassed, as he had been unwilling to come, not knowing where she was taking him. He had forgotten and couldn't visualise the Group, despite her trying to tell him repeatedly. She mentioned that he enjoyed himself when he was there, as he loved playing snooker and socialising with the other men, but it was always a battle to leave the house. I suggested that she get a snooker cue (or ask a friend or family member to get one for him) and when it was time to get ready to go, she could bring it out to act as a visual prompt to remind him where he was going.

Recognising people is often easier than remembering names and words.

Sometimes you can help your partner remember by using pictures as well as props. Remember that all of your senses may be able to help: sight, hearing, touch, smell and taste. We communicate in so many ways, and not just through the words that we speak.

'A man does not consist of memory alone. He has feeling, will, sensibility, moral being ... It is here ... you may touch him, and see a profound change.'

– Dr. Alexander R. Luria

Movement can help us remember, such as moving to music and dancing. If possible, you may think about joining a Tai Chi or yoga class. Encourage your partner to clap to the rhythm, this can help them focus their attention. Be mindful that if your partner's mobility and movement is affected, particularly if they have Lewy body dementia or Parkinson's disease dementia, you may need to consider chair movements.

Recent research has shown that some people who have mild to moderate dementia may be able to learn new things and be able to aid their memories with help. This is called cognitive rehabilitation. By rehearsing and using strategies such as mnemonics (a pattern of letters, or associations such as using a rhyme), remembering numbers by chunking them (where there is a long number to remember, chunk it into threes e.g. 123 456 789) and using memory aids, your partner may be able to improve their concentration and attention*. But be aware that this could also lead to further stress and pressure for them, be mindful about whether or not this will help them feel better.

Some types of dementia can affect our knowing where we are in time and place quite early on in the condition and can cause much worry if the person tends to go out alone (see chapter six and nine for further tips and advice). There are many products on the market that may help prompt the memory and help with orientation with the use of technology. This is known as assistive technology. These include talking clocks, watches, medication dispensers, alarm timers and message players to use as reminders. Audible alarms may be used as alerts and reminders for your partner such as a simple alarm clock, watch or mobile phone that may help remind them, for example, that it is time to eat. If your partner has a tendency to forget to take important medication, visual and audible medication dispensers can also help.

Day-to-day routines are highly recommended, place visible reminders of what is going to happen and where you are going around your home. Choose a place in the home (such as near the front door or in the kitchen) where you can put up a white board for messages, shopping lists, calendars, and post-it notes in a prominent

---

* http://tactustherapy.com/spaced-retrieval-training-memory/

place. Where possible, keep a diary or notebook to write things down. A large plain clock may help your partner with their idea of time (If they struggle to read the clock it may be worth trying a digital one). Get someone to help you pre- programme important numbers into your phone and put up a list of emergency phone numbers on your whiteboard (this will help you both).

_____

"We use chalk boards at home for my Mum: they seem less business-like and clinical. Often my kids will draw pictures on them to depict the thing we want my Mum to remember."

– Suzy

_____

If your partner continues to use the phone, consider buying one with push buttons, large numbers and a photograph of the person next to their pre-programmed number. Speak to your telephone provider about the services they offer, for example when you are out of the house you may wish your home phone to be diverted to your mobile.

Try and have one place for keeping keys, glasses and money, a large bowl may be a good idea here, but if your partner tends to lose important items such as keys, purse/wallet or phone, you could consider buying an object locator. This is a gadget that can be attached to the item and when a remote control (labelled) is pressed, it sets off a beeping noise. Be mindful that some of these products can be expensive; make sure you have a family member and/or health and social care professional to help you make your choices and choose a reputable source whether on the internet or on the high street. Another good idea is to give a trusted neighbour or relative a spare key in the event of loss.

Put pictures on cupboard doors to show what is behind the door, such as a picture of a cup and saucer on a kitchen cupboard door. I have known some people to actually take the doors off. You may also want to put a picture up on your partner's bedroom door or hang a familiar piece of clothing there to remind them where their room is.

Happy memories can be stimulated when looking through photographs, watching films, listening to music, sharing food, or touching objects such as souvenirs, shells and gardening implements (see chapter four). Try to avoid becoming isolated and don't give up on the enjoyable things you have done together. There may still be ways to participate, whether it is singing, dancing, art groups, or seeing friends at the local café or pub. Being physically and socially active can have a great effect on memory and most places have community services which offer stimulating activities. Local libraries may be a good place to start.

"We may be confined nowadays, more confined now, but I don't wander off, but there are times when we used to strike out...you need the memories when you can't strike out...although we strike out to the Forget Me Not club."

– Bill

I hope you have found this chapter helpful in explaining about how your partner's memory can be affected and how this may make them feel. By following the practical ideas, you will help them feel less stressed and overcome some of the difficulties they experience. In doing so, these suggestions should help you both reconnect together in your everyday lives.

SUMMARY OF CHAPTER THREE

How dementia can affect memory

- Short term memory loss causes difficulty in accomplishing tasks and creates repetitive language and behaviour
- The ability to concentrate is affected
- Over time longer term memories such as remembering names and faces can be affected
- Orientation to time of day and place can become muddled

Approaches to help with memory

- Help to relax, avoid stress
- Use eye contact and speak slowly
- Use the senses – seeing, hearing, tasting, touching, smelling, movement
- Break down instructions into chunks
- Label doors with pictures of what is behind them
- Use highly visible lists, calendars, post it notes
- Consider assistive technology
- Keep important objects such as keys in a designated place
- Stick to a routine
- Try some meaningful reminiscence of happy events and make use of the senses
- Join a group (e.g. memory café, singing group, etc.)

NOTES

Date:	Comment:

Write specific strategies here that help your partner with their memory.

NOTES

Date: Comment:

NOTES

Date:	Comment:

NOTES

Date:	Comment:

CHAPTER FOUR

Staying Connected through Life Stories

How to re-connect by creating your life stories that you can enjoy together

The stories we love best live in us forever.

JK ROWLING

We all have a story to tell about our lives and sometimes we enhance them with funny anecdotes, which, over time can feel more like fact to us the more we recall them. In the end, what really happened and what we remember happening may be very different. But does this really matter? Our memories for events in our lives are coloured by those we spent time with. Our families, friends, what we were doing, work, social life, the fashion, music and politics of the day etc. Even though we may have some similarities with people of our own age who may have shared common experiences, our specific stories are our own. Sometimes where the facts become hazy, the emotions attached to memories are still very real. Happy, sad, angry, joyful – everyone will have experienced strong memories in relation to certain life events. Perhaps the birth of a child, school life, university or a first job, engagement and wedding, death of a loved one, anniversaries and holidays. Our lives are multi-coloured with feelings.

This is the same for those people who are living with dementia. One great way to keep a connection together is to work on your life stories together. Get out your photographs, certificates, ornaments or souvenirs, just as we created scrap books when we were younger.

"I feel quite happy about these things; I can remember the times I had but not the names...sometimes I'm fed up when I can't remember but I still like going through these."

– Marjorie

You may wish to start by drawing a timeline that show all the significant stages of yours and your partner's life and transitions. Get a large blank sheet of paper or use the page at the end of this chapter and draw a long line. Start with birth going through childhood, onto adulthood to the present day. You can include names of schools and dates, names of places, jobs, wedding days, birth of children and grandchildren. Or you can choose a theme, such as holidays, hobbies, family life or jobs, and bring together all the things that you can find around the home that are relevant to this. You may wish to paste photographs on the timeline and put it up on your wall for your partner to see every day.

Get a scrapbook, or if you're more technologically savvy, you can create a digital timeline and lifestory so that you have a document that expresses the key moments and people in your partner's life. Photographs are helpful here (do this for yourself too). As mentioned in chapter one, it would be a great way to involve families and friends as they can often feel unsure about how to help. Keeping them in contact with your partner will also help prevent your partner from solely relying on you.

Be mindful of any painful memories that are best avoided, although you do need to be aware of significant occasions throughout your partner's life that may start to trouble them now. When creating a lifestory, it is usually best to focus on the positive occasions and memories.

"Of course, the things that we are talking about now are the happy ones, there are other memories that will block up, not block but come up and they are not good; take them out and look at them and hopefully put them back, but I'd say they are a part of you."

– Gerry

A lifestory in book form accompanied by props you can touch, such as tools or materials provides prompts and information that may help your partner connect with you and others around them. Within the lifestory, add some smells, such as an oily rag for car enthusiasts, flowers, polish or perfume or anything that may evoke positive memories. Create a memory box or rummage box to keep these things together. If your partner has a keen interest in sport you may wish to include some sporting memorabilia*.

One of the first things you can start doing now is to get out the photographs together and sit down with a cuppa and enjoy spending the time together. Often when we are in the midst of caring we are so busy *doing,* that we stop *being.* Sometimes we have to stop and just spend time together enjoying each other's company. Think of using all of your senses to help.

"I found I was so tired and fed up of all the hard work, I started feeling angry and resentful when she didn't respond and then the guilt would sink in. When I heard about lifestories, I thought, I haven't got the energy for this. But I found myself slowing picking up things around the home and putting them together in a shoebox for her to sort out. We were both keen gardeners; I went to the old greenhouse and brought in some packets of seeds and her trug. Sometimes she just sits and shows no interest and

---

other days she fiddles about with them. I have learned that it doesn't matter if she forgets to put the seeds in the pots of compost anymore – she enjoys the feel and smell of the soil although I have to make sure that she doesn't try to eat it. Sometimes I'll bring in a plate of cherry tomatoes and we enjoy these together. I don't know if she remembers that we used to grow them, but I do and it brings me some joy in remembering what we used to do together."

– Amar

Remember, when going through your photo albums together, the facts of the names of places, people and times aren't necessarily important, as these memories may not come easily. While it is important for you to mention these, don't try to test their memory. The memories of feelings and emotions stay around for much, much longer than memories of facts such as names of people and places. Focus more on the feelings.

Bear in mind whether your partner can see the photos easily: make sure there is plenty of light, and if they wear glasses, make sure they are clean. Sometimes people can have difficulty with their vision due to age and the dementia, so a trip to the optician is important. You may want to get some family members and friends to help by getting photographs enlarged to a bigger size and laminate them, or getting them digitalised so that you can view them on a large screen, maybe as a film show. Think of their hearing as well; make sure that if they wear a hearing aid, the ear isn't blocked with wax, the hearing aid is in and switched on with the battery working.

Do you have any music that would go with your memories? (see Chapter Two)

"I have seen deeply demented patients weep or shiver as they listen to music they have never heard before, and I think they can experience the entire range of feelings the rest of us can, and that dementia, at least at these times, is no bar to emotional depth. Once one has seen such responses, one knows that there is still a self to be called upon, even if music, and only music, can do the calling."

– Dr. Oliver Sacks

Go back to your playlists (Chapter Two). Music can have a fantastic effect; put it on, and you may find yourself dancing again (dancing in the chair can also be great if you are a little unsteady), and certainly singing together can create a great feeling (none of us remember all of the words, so that doesn't matter). Rhythm and movement, even if it is a foot tapping, can really help us to connect at a deep level.

During a reminiscence session, a spouse told me that her husband could not communicate anymore, to the point of her saying that he was not himself anymore, it was as if he had left his body and that he would not respond in any way, not a flicker. She was understandably very distressed by this. We watched an old film with a Humphrey Littleton jazz soundtrack for the group. I noticed that as the soundtrack started, his shoulders relaxed very slightly, his foot started tapping very gently and a slight smile came across his face. These changes were very subtle but they showed that he was responding. His wife went home and dug out all their old jazz records, it gave her some hope that he was still there and that she could find a way to connect with him.

Sometimes we need to look for the subtlest of signs to see a response, but in the midst of caring, it is so easy to miss because we are so tired and often stressed. Thinking about the senses is a great start. You may have old film footage of family holidays that might be pleasurable to watch or may be able to buy DVDs of holiday places, favourite films, memorable sports events and comedy that will help you and your partner stay connected with meaningful memories.

While some senses may be impaired or might have changed since the dementia, it is worth thinking about how each one may help, either on their own or mixed together, such as taste and smell. When you can find time, or ask a family member, get some ice cream or food and drinks that have a connection with your memories (maybe a picnic hamper). This may be a good approach if your partner is sometimes reluctant to eat or drink. Bringing food into the context of a happy memory such as a picnic can be a helpful approach to eating and drinking (see Chapter Seven). We all love to reminisce and feel nostalgic, so give it a try. This can also be done with other family members, friends or caregivers/befrienders whilst you have a rest.

Touch is a very important sense. The feel of a favourite piece of clothing, patchwork cushions, the texture of a favourite jacket or the touch of objects such as sea shells, sand, buttons, grass, jewellery, tools; material helps to reconnect with the outside world and can usually stimulate feelings. Having rummage boxes filled with such objects around the house can help avoid frustrations when your partner may have lost some of their possessions. Think about the things your partner would have used in their day-to-day lives, maybe related to hobbies, school or work (for example, tools, wool, textiles, car parts, paints, sports equipment such as a leather football, tennis racquet, cricket bat, hockey stick). Make sure they are associated with good memories and avoid sharp objects.

Some people find the touch of soft toys, dolls and pets comforting". Clay making can be an extremely enjoyable pastime that can help your partner with their fine motor skills and give them a sense of creativity and achievement. Don't worry if it's a bit messy, get involved in it, you may be surprised at what you can achieve together and have fun in the meantime.

Involve younger family members and friends. When

" https://www.dementiauk.org/the-use-of-dolls-in-dementia-care/

creating a lifestory, they will learn a lot about your partner's life and be able to share the past while enjoying the moment together in the present. If you are reading this as a friend of somebody who has dementia, ask them or their partner what would be the best thing you could do to help. It may just be spending a few moments together to be there and listen or it may be helpful to be involved in some of these activities.

"I didn't know that my Grampy had been a great dancer and he and my Nan had won many competitions. I really enjoyed getting their rosettes, medals and photos together with my Nan. I realise that they liked the same things that I do now."

– Nia

Sometimes friends can slip away, which can be very upsetting. This is often because they do not know what to do, what to say or how to respond. By involving them with practical things like helping to gather information together, they can contribute to your partner's lifestory. This will help them realise that they have a part to play, feel more confident and be in a better position to help and stay connected with you both.

A document of your partner's lifestory will also be of enormous help if they have to go into hospital or move into residential care, or if you have caregivers/befrienders coming into your home. By making sure you have important information on hand about your partner's life and current likes and dislikes you will help others communicate and connect with them when they may have difficulty expressing themselves.

I hope that you have found this chapter helpful in showing you how you can use your senses to help remember positive memories and by being involved in activities together can be enjoyable while helping keep you and your partner connected in meaningful ways.

SUMMARY OF CHAPTER FOUR

How dementia can affect a person's memory

- Memories for facts such as names, dates and places can fade
- Emotions attached to memories stay around for much longer
- The senses may help stimulate memories

How to help create lifestories

- Involve families and friends in helping chart important aspects of your loved one's life
- Draw a timeline with events such as marriage, birth of children, first job, hobbies, holidays

- Get a scrapbook together & memory box to include meaningful objects
- Focus on positive memories while being mindful about any traumatic past life events
- Remember to involve all the senses (where possible) to explore things that are meaningful in one's life
  - Visual – Use of photographs, films, souvenirs
  - Hearing – Music- create a playlist of favourite music, sounds such as birdsong, transport etc
  - Taste – Incorporate foods associated with memories into a reminiscence moment
  - Smell – Very powerful in evoking memories, try perfumes, favourite hair products, get outside and smell the grass, flowers
  - Touch – Use materials such as wool, button boxes, tools, wood
  - Movement – Encourage with music and sound, foot tapping, rocking, dancing (where possible), hand movements

NOTES

_Draw a timeline here or make notes about specific
people, places, events and memories that you
want to include in your partner's lifestory._

NOTES

NOTES

NOTES

NOTES

CHAPTER FIVE

Creating a Calm, Safe Home

How to help your care partner feel content and safe at home

Home is where you feel at home and are treated well.
DALAI LAMA

People living with dementia often fare best in surroundings that are familiar to them. The home environment can provide a sense of security, and this can help to maintain a feeling of confidence as our homes often reflect a sense of who we are. You may improve each other's wellbeing and decrease the risk of confusion and potential falls when focusing on creating a place of calmness at home. In fact, Florence Nightingale wrote much about the importance of environment for healing and caring, which included natural light, warmth, fresh air and good diet. It is important to get outdoors and socialise as much as possible too, for yourself and your partner. Pets can also be a great source of comfort. Don't forget to involve any family and friends and let them read this book too.

But try not to make too many changes to the feel of your home, only make alterations that will help towards your partner's independence, safety and contentment. If they live on their own, consider exploring assistive technology to help them keep their independence while making sure they are safe at home.

"He still cooks for himself and I don't want him thinking I am fussing too much, but I am still his Mum! I'm afraid he may one day forget to turn the gas off. I worry all the time because he has no one with him throughout the day and night."

– Jean (age 92)

Once again, assistive technology may help, such as fitting automatic cut-out systems to turn off the gas supply on cookers and fires after a specified time. If you have a microwave, make sure all metal containers and pans are kept out of sight. I would strongly advise making sure that your home has temperature, smoke and carbon monoxide alarms. You may be able to speak to your local fire service to see if they can provide any help and support. In some cases, they will fit alarms for you. Failing that, speak to your doctor or health and social care professional for some advice. Water and flood detectors may help where taps have been left on. If your partner is a smoker it would be worth putting a drop of water in the bottom of their ashtray to reduce the risk of fire. You may also consider using special covers for electrical power points/outlets.

People who have dementia may have difficulty with their eyesight, whether it is failing sight or the dementia is affecting how they see (visual perception). They may also have problems with walking, tending to shuffle more, and will therefore be at risk of falling. You may need to consider getting a strong chair with armrests that should help them sit down and stand up more easily.

Make sure your home is light, making full use of natural light, and try to avoid shadows. Be aware that patterned carpets and wallpaper may appear confusing. Sometimes where there are patterns or mats, the person may be confused by what they see such as thinking the rug is a hole in the floor and may be fearful of stepping into it. Shiny floors may appear wet and slippery to your partner. Where there is a difference between flooring between rooms, your partner may see it as a step, so be aware that they may feel the need to step up over a line between carpets/flooring or not wish to step over at all.

"It seemed to happen quite suddenly but Bill didn't want to come into the kitchen. It didn't make sense: he seemed to stop right at the doorway and wouldn't go any further. I took him by the hand but he still wouldn't budge an inch. I got so frustrated with him and felt terrible after I shouted at him. The nurse then told me that he might not recognise the strip of flooring between the hall and the kitchen. My daughter helped us get a carpet fitter to change the flooring and make it plain and the same colour throughout the downstairs. Now Bill has no trouble and I've been told is less likely to fall as he shuffles, as the flooring is all one colour and the same material. It made sense to me once I knew why and makes his and my life easier."

– Hilary

Remove rugs, as they can cause falls. Make distinctions between walls and floors. I have some experience of this personally.

One day at the opticians, my glasses were taken from me (I am extremely short-sighted!) and I was asked to sit on the chair. I nearly fell on the floor because the chairs and the floor were the same colour: I couldn't tell what was the floor and what was the chair. It certainly made me feel a bit frightened and vulnerable.

This can often be the case for the person who has dementia, who may see things differently. Remember that what they are seeing is very real to them and may be different from what you see. The person who has dementia may even have difficulty recognising their own face in the mirror and become troubled by this.

"Jackie started getting really upset when she looked in the bathroom mirror. She started shouting at herself and pointing angrily. It took me ages to realise that she didn't recognise herself. The nurse told me that she might not recognise herself, as she may remember a younger version of her face. It broke my heart. Is this really what can happen? I realised it was better to get rid of the mirror, but I still needed to shave. In the end I fitted a blind over it and kept it covered when she was in the bathroom and rolled it up when I needed to use it."

– David

Your partner may also have difficulty distinguishing between light switches and the walls and toilet seats and the floors, so it is a good idea to try to create a contrast of colours. For instance, if the light switch is white, the wall needs to be a different colour. Toilet seats need to contrast against the floor and the wall. In fact, you can actually buy toilet seats that glow in the dark that may help if your partner needs to go in the night. It is also a good idea to keep the toilet door open so that your partner can see where they need to go and it may act as a prompt for them.

Try to create a calm environment by clearing clutter and making the most of natural light. Open the curtains and if you have a pleasant outlook make the most of it. If your partner struggles with the reflection in the window, it might be worth buying some very fine net curtains that reduce it but still show the view.

Relaxing music and plants can be helpful in creating a sense of calmness and healing. Be aware that if there is background noise from a TV, computer or radio, you may be competing with it when trying to have a conversation. When speaking with your partner, turn off all extraneous noise to give them full opportunity to hear what you are saying. Remember, they may not always be able to understand the words that you are saying and need time to gather their thoughts and speech. Focus on just 'being' with your partner and not always 'doing', thereby *Finding the Light* within. If your partner moves into residential care or with a family member, it is important to provide a sense of familiarity to help them to feel safe. (see Chapter Twelve)

"When Mum moved in with us, I wanted her to feel comfortable with her familiar things around her. I gave her the choice of where she wanted to put her crockery in the kitchen. She naturally chose a cupboard that seemed right for her. Maybe this was because it was in the same position as hers in her own kitchen."

– Suzy

By keeping meaningful objects around your partner you can help them feel secure and safe.

"One of the most important things when Mum moved in with us was her bedside cabinet and all that it contained.

We made sure that her lamp and clock sat on the top in the same position as they had done for the past thirty years, stretching back to when she would get me up for school in the mornings!! She also had a favourite knitted toy that had always sat on top of the clock. I didn't know what it was – from as far back as I can remember it had always been there, but I had never asked her about it. I later found out that she bought it as a souvenir on honeymoon. We never move it, we always keep it in the same position. We did this so even if Mum didn't know where she was or why she was there, she would feel some sense of familiarity when waking up and going to sleep."

– Suzy

Sometimes we may not know the significance of objects, clothes and things or the stories behind them. Try to find out when working together on your lifestories. You could also label your photographs of families and friends around the home (refer to chapter four; timeline) saying what their relationship is to you and your partner.

When it comes to feeling safe at home, you may also want to prevent nuisance cold callers or sales people coming to your door, sending you emails, or contacting you by post/mail and phone. Unfortunately, some people take advantage of those who are vulnerable and try to sell them things that they do not need or even try to fraudulently extort money (this is called scamming). Some local authorities provide stickers to put on your windows and doors to help dissuade such people. As mentioned in chapter one, it is worth considering blocking your phone number and email address to unknown callers and cancelling unwanted mail/post that comes to your door*. If your loved one lives on their own you may want to change their front door lock to a key safe system. This is a small box that has a code that allows only those who have the password access to their key.

If you have a garden, try and both spend time outside together, ask your family and friends to make sure that any trip hazards are reduced such as making sure that paths aren't slippery, recoiling water hoses and cutting back overgrown plants. Planting herbs can provide lovely scents, whilst being safe to eat. If you have a shed or a garage, it is a great place to putter about and let your partner be engaged in some activity but make sure that any toxic substances and hazards are removed.

You may want to put together some boxes of objects in the garden to help your partner stay interested and occupied, such as a woodwork, gardening, motor, textile or tools (see chapter four). If your partner has a tendency to wander and you are concerned for their safety you may need to camouflage any gates with plants and paint and put a bench in the middle of your garden as a point of interest. You could pop a box of objects on the bench that might occupy your partner's time and possibly stop them from walking away from the home

---

* http://www.ageuk.org.uk/Documents/EN-GB/Information-guides/AgeUKIG05_
Avoiding_scams_inf.pdf?epslanguage=en-GB?dtrk=true

or garden. Make any pathways circular so that they lead back to the house.

It is hard to come to terms with how the dementia may affect your partner. Be mindful that they may not experience all the things mentioned here. Your goal is to help them and yourself to be as content as possible and your awareness of how dementia may affect them, will help both of you. I hope that by reading this chapter you have learned about the small (and maybe larger) changes you can make to your home that will help you both. When creating a calmer environment in your home you may find the space to keep or find your connection together once more.

SUMMARY OF CHAPTER FIVE

How dementia can create safety concerns

- Eyesight and visual perception is often affected which may affect what or how your partner is seeing
- Movement and mobility may change, such as shuffling when walking
- Judgement and reasoning around risk and safety may change

Approaches to help with creating a calm safe home

- Familiarity can lead to a greater sense of security
- Familiar pets can be comforting
- Avoid clutter
- Make use of natural light to help with eyesight
- Make distinctions between floors, walls and chairs
- Remove rugs
- Shiny floors may be seen as slippery
- Contrast colours for light switches, toilets, walls & floors
- Try and avoid patterns and shadows
- Create calmness with plants, colours & gentle music
- Keep meaningful objects in sight
- Plant herbs in the garden
- Make sure hazards are reduced in the garden
- Create a central point of interest in the garden such as a bench or shed with rummage boxes
- Make sure paths are circular allowing for a return to the house

NOTES

Write a list of changes you could make in your home or a plan for others to help you with.

NOTES

NOTES

NOTES

CHAPTER SIX

Sleep is the Best Medication

*Gentle approaches to help
you both feel rested*

*Sleep is the golden chain that ties health
and our bodies together.*

THOMAS DEKKER

Sleep and knowing where you are in time and place can often be affected by dementia, particularly for those who have Lewy body dementia and Parkinson's disease dementia. This can often result in your partner sleeping more in the day and being restless at night. Some people may become more agitated around late afternoon and at night-time (this is called "sundowning") and they may become more disoriented if they sleep in the day; confusing dreams with reality.

"I was so tired with him waking me up and wandering in the night, I didn't feel that I could go on any more. Until I realised, he'd been napping in the chair for most of the day! When we had a befriender to help, she would go for a walk with him, they chatted about his love of steam trains and he seemed much happier when he came back, and I'm sure it helped him have a better night's sleep. It doesn't always work but I feel a bit better now too."

– Nas

It is important to try to maintain the natural rhythms of day and night, maximising the use of daylight. Where possible, go out for a walk together in the day or ask a friend or befriender to go for a walk with your partner. Try to go outdoors into nature, as this can help you both become more in-tune with the natural rhythms of your environment. Being outside in natural daylight is one of the most important cues that help the brain distinguish between night and day. Don't forget to be aware of your senses. Feeling a breeze on your skin, seeing a view, touching the bark of a tree, smelling freshly cut grass, hearing birdsong, a river flowing or sounds of the sea, touching the earth and sand can help you both feel re-connected and give you a sense of wellbeing. If you live in a city and cannot get to the countryside easily, find a local park. You will notice that by getting outdoors, you will feel more connected with the world and less likely to feel lonely and isolated. Don't forget, if it is difficult to encourage your partner to go out, show them some photographs or props that may help. If you cannot get outdoors, help them sit close to a window for their brain to register as much natural light as possible. You may want to talk to your doctor about bright white light therapy that has been known to help some people who have dementia over a period of time. Being exposed to morning light has been known to help a person feel less agitated and where possible if you can get out together in the morning you may find that both your night's sleep improves.

When at home try listening to the sounds of nature on a CD or on the computer: this could include bird-song and the sounds of the sea and will bring the natural world to you. If you are unable to go out, ask your family and friends to bring you some flowers or plants to have around your home.

While an afternoon nap can be a good relaxing habit, too much sleep in the day will upset the person's body clock even more, so try to keep this short. Social, mental and physical activities can be helpful in keeping your partner engaged throughout the day, which may stop them sleeping.

"We often took the residents out for a trip on the local canal barge in the Brecon Beacons National Park, followed by a cream tea. On leaving the Home, all would climb aboard the bus, often forgetting where they were going. But there was always a sense of excitement and anticipation. On returning, they had clearly enjoyed the day and were all chatting together, many not remembering where they had been or what they had done. But they were happy socialising together and had a change of scenery. The night staff reported that their sleep patterns settled and most of them slept throughout the night for a whole week after the adventure!"

– Rita, Care Home Nurse Manager

As well as socialising outside the house (where possible), think about how your partner can stay occupied and stimulated when at home. Maybe play some games together. Remember, the facts of the games don't matter; the engagement that you have when being together may offer some mental and sociable stimulation and prevent too much daytime napping.

"My daughter brought my little grandson over one afternoon and he lay on the floor colouring, drawing and playing with his toy cars. I couldn't believe my eyes – Ted got down on all fours and started colouring with him and picking up the cars, rubbing the wheels against the palm of his hand. We had some difficulty getting him up, but we moved the cars and the crayons onto the kitchen table, where they both sat all afternoon. They didn't say a word, just drew and ran the cars over the table. That is the first interest that Ted has shown in anything for the past year and a half. I've now turned our dining room table into an art room and some days Ted will sit there and draw, especially when our grandson visits, other times he stares into space but it keeps him awake in the day. I'm sure this has helped him sleep better at night."

– Joan

Research now shows that being involved in creative pursuits can help the person who has dementia and the people around them in a number of ways. Get out pens, paints, crayons, clay and pencils and try some shared art together, jigsaws can be good. Where possible ask a family member to join you so they can help you clear up afterwards. You may be surprised at what can be created and how you can connect together, where you can, involve the children. Be in the moment. There are some great mindfulness colouring books in the shops now, although it is good to try some freedom of expression. It is important to realise that the end result is not as important as the actual process of the activity. Try out new things, and keep an open mind to what you could both enjoy. Keeping your partner and yourself involved in activities helps to keep up interest and stimulation and may help you both to get a better night's sleep and stop dozing too much throughout the day. Create a daytime schedule that includes mealtimes within the routine. The use of a large clock may help your partner to understand what time of day it is.

When considering sleep, it is important to remember what their preferences were before they developed dementia, if they were used to sleeping in a double bed they may find that being in a single bed now feels too small. Did they like a hard or soft bed and pillows? I would, however, recommend putting the bed next to a wall if they are at risk of falling out. Try to maintain a regular wake-up time, and at bedtime, reduce the noise level in the house, as too much sensory stimulation can be confusing. Limit screen time for a couple of hours before bedtime. It is wise not to use a computer, tablet or phone at least two hours before bedtime as it has been found that these screens in particular, can detrimentally affect natural sleep.

Eat the evening meal at least an hour before bedtime and play a quiet piece of relaxing music before going to bed. Over time, there may be an association between the music and bed, just like a lullaby. Try three drops of Lavender in the room (but don't use too much as this can have an opposite effect, also be mindful if certain scents act as triggers to changes in how your partner responds). Remove all daytime clothing and avoid bright colours in the bedroom. Use of dark curtains in the bedroom can be helpful, but be aware that if your partner does get up at night, a light with a movement sensor could be arranged to minimise the risk of falling (assistive technology). You could also try putting reflective tape along the wall to direct them to the toilet. Failing that, a commode by the bedside may be helpful if your partner wakes up needing to go to the toilet.

Assistive technology can provide motion sensors to alert you when your partner may wander at night[*]. Some motion sensors can monitor movement between rooms and certain times and trigger an alarm on your mobile

---

[*] https://www.alzheimers.org.uk/info/20091/what_we_think/85/assistive_technology
http://www.alzra.org/eldercare/assistive-technology/
https://www.dementia.org.au/information/resources/more-resources/assistive-technology

phone, so they may give you peace of mind if your partner lives alone. If they tend to wake and wander at night they may be in pain or may be hungry or thirsty but are unable to tell you. There is nothing wrong with a little midnight feast if it helps! Stewed apple may be a naturally sweet treat that is soft to eat. If they are in pain or discomfort it is worth speaking to your doctor. Some pain killing medications can be given in the form of creams and skin patches.

Don't expect miraculous changes overnight, but by creating a routine and considering the above approaches, your partner's sleep pattern may settle with time.

Unfortunately, sleep can be affected by the physical changes in the brain in those who have dementia and if you try these strategies and your partner is still restless at night, sleep and rest when they do. Speak to your doctor if you are not getting the rest you need, you may need to consider your partner receiving temporary care for you to have a rest and help you recharge your batteries. This is known as respite care (see chapter twelve).

I hope this chapter has helped you understand how dementia affects sleep and that trying the approaches recommended may help you both get the rest you need.

SUMMARY OF CHAPTER SIX

How dementia can affect sleep

- Can affect the internal body clock, dreaming and non-dreaming sleep stages
- Increased restlessness at late afternoon – "sundowning"
- Increased daytime sleep
- Changes in sleep pattern due to dementia, ageing and /or medical conditions and medication

Approaches to help with sleep

- Maintain the natural rhythms of day and night maximising the use of natural day light
- Get outdoors (where possible), and sit close to a window
- Keep your partner occupied in creative activities throughout the day
- Keep to a regular wake up and bedtime
- Check if they are in pain or discomfort
- Check if they are hungry or thirsty
- Do they need to use the toilet? Consider a commode by the bed
- Rest & sleep when your loved one does
- Create a regular schedule throughout the day

- Speak to your doctor about bright light therapy
- Remember what your partner's preferences were before dementia
  - Size of bed
  - Temperature of room
  - Soft/hard bed, pillows
- Bedtime routine should include:
  - Eat no later than 1 hour before bed
  - Encourage use of the toilet
  - Try gentle music (lullaby) to create an association between time and bed, Lavender drops
  - Dark curtains (but be aware of risk of falls, use a light sensor for night)
  - Avoid use of Phone, computer or tablet at least 2 hours before bed.

NOTES

Date: Preferences (sleep patterns, what helps?):

Write down your partner's preferences and sleep patterns here and note what strategies may help you both be rested.

NOTES

Date: Preferences (sleep patterns, what helps?):

NOTES

Date: Preferences (sleep patterns, what helps?):

CHAPTER SEVEN

Tips for Eating and Drinking

How good nutrition and hydration can provide balance in your lives

Let food be thy medicine and medicine be thy food.
HIPPOCRATES

Nutrition is central to keeping you and your partner as healthy as possible, as well as maintaining the enjoyment of sharing food together. Dementia can considerably affect a person's association with food and drink. They may lose the ability to recognise if they are hungry or thirsty, forget to eat and drink and/or develop a "sweet tooth" with a tendency to binge. Changes in eating habits and preferences often occur with those people who have frontotemporal dementia and sometimes in those living with Alzheimer's disease. Taste buds may change over the course of a lifetime too. Just because your partner may have disliked or liked a certain food throughout their life doesn't mean that they still do. A number of problems can arise if they are not eating well. Poor diet can lead to further problems, such as low blood sugar, headaches, constipation and urinary tract infections, which can all lead to more confusion, restlessness and poor sleep.

"Trying to get Tom to drink was a nightmare: he never seemed to be thirsty. He started getting really restless and angry and I didn't know what to do with him. I managed to get the doctor to see him and he told me he had a urinary infection and that this can make him more confused. He gave me some liquid antibiotics to take (luckily, he liked the banana flavour) and told me to give him more drinks – easier said than done! From then on, I started making him banana smoothies; sometimes he likes them, other times he leaves it and I'm back to square one, but it made me realise I needed to think differently when he refuses to drink. I did try a straw but I don't think he knows how to suck the drink through it. This made me very upset but I keep trying to find ways. I realise it's better to keep trying, giving him sips every two hours helps, and then I know he's had a drink."

– **Harry**

If your loved one lives alone, it may be worth putting a clear door on their fridge and cupboards to remind them of where their food is kept.

Be aware that your partner may not be able to see the food on their plate if the food is the same colour. Try to use pattern-free plates and a contrasting colour to the food as they may have difficulty working out what is the food and what is the plate. If they have difficulty holding a fork, knife or spoon, you can buy special cutlery that is easier to grip. Try the hand over hand approach; where you hold the cutlery and they put their hand over yours, so that they continue to use their hand, feel the cutlery and sense the movement.

Other things to consider in relation to eating and drinking include making sure that you both have regular trips to the dentist as your partner may be in pain due to problems with their teeth, gums and dentures. If they wear dentures, try to make sure they continue to wear them as they may forget to put them in or forget how to wear them. Ask your dentist to mark them with their name. If possible, try to introduce an electric tooth-brush or a toothbrush with a wide handle to make gripping better.

If your partner is inactive, they may not feel like eating as much, so it is a good idea to try to keep active together, and where possible, get out and about in the fresh air and meet up with family and friends. If they are restless, they may also need some extra calories.

If you find that you are getting tired of preparing food, consider using local companies that deliver meals to your door. Where you continue to dine out, it is worth contacting the restaurant beforehand to explain your situation to the staff and to find out if they are receptive to you and your partner's needs. This will include requiring more time when choosing and eating the meal; making sure that the lighting is bright enough; providing menus with pictures and requesting a table in a more private part of the restaurant while making sure that your partner is able to see the rest of the room (so that they can work out where unfamiliar noises may be coming from). It is also worthwhile considering the noise level; carpets help to muffle sounds and background music should be kept low.

Your partner may not be able to communicate that they don't like the taste or texture of the food, so try a varied selection of small nutritious portions, just like tapas, a mezze, or buffet. It may be helpful to talk about and name the food as you are sharing it. "Good food and drink, little and often" is the best mantra. Encourage small sips of water throughout the day (and you do the same, as you can often forget about yourself when busy). Keep bowls of small healthy food around the home such as strawberries, grapes and cut up carrots. Foods high in water are good to help your partner feel nourished such as berries, watermelon and cucumber.

Be a little creative if your partner isn't keen to eat: make it an occasion, find moments in the day such as a small picnic when reminiscing over holiday photographs, or, if appropriate, use a sandwich box that's familiar to the one used when your partner was working. If possible, try going fruit picking together with family and friends, then enjoy an ice cream together when the season is right. Think about foods that are associated with happy memories of sharing. Fish and chips at the seaside, pizza, whatever you both enjoy. You may want to introduce some familiar music to go with the meal or some sound effects that remind you of those times: not too loud and distracting, but gentle and in the background.

"I used to dread mealtimes; trying to help my wife to eat was becoming more and more difficult. I am afraid to say that I sometimes lost my temper, until the memory clinic staff gave me some advice about trying finger foods and not big meals. It was easier to prepare, it made me relax more (which I'm sure helped) and sometimes we would sit all afternoon munching on bread sticks, carrots and olives. She seemed to pick at the food but I realised that she was having small amounts over time."

– Amir

The sounds of preparing food can remind us of past happy memories along with the smells associated with cooking. Try to get your partner involved in the preparation, where you have time, rolling out dough and using pastry cutters can be a great occupation that stimulates the senses. Remember that all cooking and preparation takes a number of steps (short term memory loss), so your partner may need to be reminded of some of the stages. Ask them to lay the table (it doesn't matter how it is done), being occupied helps your partner feel valued and may help towards slowing down their deterioration. Be patient with them and prompt gently when needed. Try to involve family and friends and if your partner has difficulty using cutlery, a buffet with finger food is a lovely way to overcome any difficulties experienced*. Introduce half portions if they are struggling to eat a large plate. Make it as appetising as possible using the senses; smells, colour, texture and differing tastes.

Cooking smells can help stimulate taste and a small sherry (if appropriate and check with your doctor) can act as an appetiser. Where possible try and encourage a healthy well-balanced diet of fruit and vegetables, fish, lean meat and wholegrains (Mediterranean diet). You can try new and different foods, as the palette can change, and a great way of having a healthy meal is as a smoothie or a milkshake (you can add all sorts of healthy ingredients here).

Many people who have dementia seem to develop a "sweet tooth" and others may lose their ability to feel full or despite feeling full, continue to binge eat. If you are concerned with their sugar intake consider replacing it with herbal Stevia, this is a natural product that tastes sweeter than sugar but does not raise blood sugar levels as sugar does. Make sure that you buy the naturally occurring herbal Stevia and not the processed, bleached type. It may also be worth trying to keep your partner

---

* https://www.nourishbyjaneclarke.com/

distracted with other activities (see previous chapters) to try and stop them overeating.

You may need to ask your doctor to refer you to a speech and language therapist if your partner experiences difficulties with swallowing or if they start to choke a little on their food. If they do have any swallowing or chewing difficulties, try softer food such as stewed fruit, a thick soup or scrambled egg. Make sure that your partner's mouth is moist before they eat by giving them sips of water. Speak to their doctor or dietician/nutritionist for advice. One great tip I have learned from Jane Clarke, at Nourish is to help your partner suck a small piece of chocolate. This can help relax their facial muscles and help them swallow. If you are concerned that they are losing weight or not getting enough nutrients into their diet you can add certain ingredients into their foods. This is known as fortifying foods. Unless, of course, if your partner has a tendency to binge or has diabetes.

Suggestions include adding:

- Skimmed milk powder
- Full fat milk
- Condensed milk
- Custard
- Cream
- Full fat yogurt
- Cheese
- Butter
- Cream

- Jam, honey and syrup
- Orange juice
- Ice cream

Try and eat together at the table, they may be more likely to eat the healthier foods that you are eating when you are with them. Avoid alcohol where bingeing may occur as this may impact on their insulin levels in the brain. Provide wholesome soups that may help them feel full and cut up other foods into small chunks.

If your partner lives alone, be mindful that they may have forgotten or have lost the ability to smell food that has gone bad. You may find it easier to make a large batch of soups/casseroles/stews and dish them into individual portions, keeping them in the fridge. They may also need prompts to remind them to eat, such as alarms or visual reminders around the home. Once again involve family and friends as eating and drinking are traditionally shared experiences.

I hope that this chapter has helped you understand how dementia can affect eating and drinking and that you will have learned some tips for overcoming some of the difficulties you may experience. By following some of the approaches you should be able to continue to share some happy times together while still enjoying good food and drink.

SUMMARY OF CHAPTER SEVEN

How dementia can affect eating and drinking

- Unable to recognise if hungry or thirsty
- Can forget to eat and drink
- May develop a "sweet tooth"
- Taste buds might change
- May tend to "binge" on food
- May not be able to communicate preferences
- Pain or constipation may affect appetite
- May not smell food that has gone bad

Approaches to help with eating and drinking

- Make sure oral health is good with regular visits to dentist
- Make sure dentures fit properly
- Get your partner involved in the preparation
- If they have been more active they may develop an appetite
- Make sure food is a contrast to the plate colour
- Smoothies and milkshakes
- Use plant based Stevia as an alternative to sugar for those with a "sweet tooth"
- If swallowing is difficult, try softer foods

such as scrambled egg and thick soup, add special food thickeners (speak to speech and language therapist or your doctor here for advice)
- Give a small piece of chocolate to suck to relax facial and jaw muscles if struggling to swallow
- Fortify foods with full fat ingredients (unless overweight, have diabetes or tend to binge)
- Make food appetising by:
  - Small appetising portions & snacks
  - Regular sips of drinks
  - Buffets & finger foods
  - Try creative approaches such as picnics, connect food to meaningful memories
  - Make batches of wholesome soups/casseroles/stews and pour into individual containers

NOTES

Date: Likes: Dislikes:

_Write down your partner's likes and dislikes
here; or what works best and what to avoid
(bearing in mind that this may change)._

NOTES

Date:	Likes:	Dislikes:

NOTES

Date: Likes: Dislikes:

NOTES

Date:	Likes:	Dislikes:

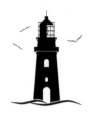

CHAPTER EIGHT

I am still me!

How to maintain your partner's dignity and help with their appearance

> *It is an absolute human certainty that no one can know his own beauty or perceive a sense of his own worth until it has been reflected back to him in the mirror of another loving, caring human being.*

JOSEPH JOHN POWELL

Appearance and personal care can often define who we are and help with our self-esteem and wellbeing. We all feel better when we have had our hair cared for and are wearing our favourite choice of clothes. Dementia can have an impact on a person's motivation, mood, understanding, memory and how they express themselves. This can affect their ability to attend to their appearance and personal care. They may start wearing the same clothes each day, be reluctant to change them and forget to wash, clean their teeth, shave or use make-up. Your partner may be unable to recognise that they need help with washing, bathing and dressing and resist help. Help them to continue with dressing independently for as long as possible, they may just need some encouragement. If your partner resists your help, it may be for all sorts of reasons, such as feeling embarrassed or exposed, not understanding what is happening or what they need to do and/or feeling a sense of loss of control.

The first thing to bear in mind is to choose the best time of day to approach personal care and be aware of potential triggers that might make your partner resistant to help. Make sure that you have plenty of time, show patience and avoid rushing them. When you decide that you do not have to rush, you can start to feel more relaxed yourself, which may help your partner feel more settled. Start off with making the bathroom a warm and relaxing one (avoiding electricity and water!) add some soft towels and if possible use three drops of Lavender essential oil in some warm water.

Let your partner do as much as they can for themselves. It is important for them to feel a sense of control and keep their independence for as long as possible. Recent research has shown that helping the person continue with well-practised tasks and avoiding taking over but giving gentle prompts, may slow down the deterioration caused by the dementia.

Remember, as their short-term memory is affected, they may need prompts at each stage. You could stick pictures of clothes on drawers and wardrobes to show them where their belongings are. Give them choices (but not too many, as that can lead to difficulties with making decisions). If your partner is struggling, avoid taking over, but offer your help and support, chat to them about what you are doing in a gentle voice and try to work co-operatively with them.

Explain all along what you want them to do or what help you are trying to give them. Give encouragement but be aware of your tone of voice; avoid sounding patronising. Talk positively about their appearance. If needed, demonstrate what you want them to do. For instance, dampen a facecloth and mime washing your own face. Think about their routines around washing and dressing. Do they have favourite products and scents? Remember how powerful our sense of smell can be.

Look for signs of needing to use the toilet. A raised toilet seat may make it easier for them to sit down (speak to your doctor). Be aware of their physical condition: are they in pain? Refer to Chapter Two for help and tips about how communication can help you find out if there is anything wrong. Make sure their dignity is preserved by helping them cover their body with a towel or a specialist washing poncho to avoid them feeling exposed.

They may not be able to use a tap so easily anymore, make sure they are clearly labelled red for hot and blue for cold as these colours are often deeply embedded in our memories. You may also need to reduce the temperature of the hot taps in your home. If your partner is reluctant to wash their hands before meals or after the toilet, give them an anti-bacterial wipe: they may copy you if you have one yourself. Where possible, it is better to be able to soak hands in water and use a favourite smelling soap. Soaking hands will help soften nails in readiness for trimming and can be quite therapeutic. You may want to fill a bowl with water and soap and put in props for your partner to rummage through, such as some small dishes, or let them see it as a hobby where objects may need cleaning. For nails, use a proper nail clipper, demonstrating on your own nails first.

For feet, you could try a foot spa. Once again, involve your partner in using it, putting your feet in first. Make sure that you are not rushed for time, as this can create a sense of anxiety. I'd recommend speaking to your doctor about arranging for a podiatrist or chiropodist to help trim their toe nails. This is particularly important if they have a physical condition that may affect their circulation (such as diabetes).

If they are having a bath or shower, avoid slippery oils, check the temperature of the water with your elbow to make sure it is not too hot or cold and use a non-slip mat inside the bath. In this instance, it may be better to use one that is the same colour as the bath, as a different colour may be seen as a hole and depth of water may not be accurately judged. Ask your family and friends to help you install a bath seat that fits across and can help where your partner may struggle to get in and out. If the soap gets too slippery put it into a stocking. Try to avoid too much steam as this may make your partner feel a little disoriented.

"Bathing can be a bit of a challenge, which I find hard, as David was fastidious about washing before the dementia. I've learnt to approach him in a different way, as I'd just get him all wound up, I would feel exhausted and upset and still he wouldn't have had a wash. I take a deep breath before I start and put on some of his favourite music in the bedroom. I try to dance with him in time to the music, moving into the bathroom, sometimes it works and sometimes it doesn't. If it doesn't, I leave it and think I'll try again later. I've made up a box of his toiletries, brushes and cufflinks to rummage through. We take the tops off the bottles and smell them, and then when he is enjoying the smell, I try to give him a wash with a warm flannel. It's not always easy but since I take my time I think he gets less wound up too."

– Joan

Creating a calming environment will help you relax together more. Be aware that your partner may not recognise things or may have visual difficulties in the bathroom. Strips of dark tape on the top sides of the bath may help to guide. Make sure you have everything to hand before you start. Avoid triggers that might cause upset, such as splashing water. Give your partner choices; is there a familiar soap smell that may help? If they don't like a shower, try a wash down. You might like to hand a cloth and prompt them, saying 'Here is the cloth, can you wash your face?' while demonstrating or miming to back up the words spoken. Make sure their skin is dried, gently taking care to note sensitive areas.

Safety-wise, make sure that your partner cannot lock themselves in the bathroom and keep cleaning products out of sight, as they may have difficulty reading or understanding the labels. Keep all electrical items away from water, as they may also have forgotten about safety hazards.

Speak to your doctor about an occupational therapy referral for grab rails, shower seats and raised toilet seats. Remove any waste bins that may be mistaken for the toilet. Where your partner is male, you could add colour to the toilet water to allow them to see where to aim more clearly. You may be able to prevent accidents if you introduce a routine for going to the toilet, such as going before or after meals.

"I found that lately I seem to mime what I want Mum to do, whether it's cleaning her teeth, washing her hands or the rest of her body. We have a bit of a laugh. I've turned into a bit of a clown sometimes, but it makes us both feel better than when I used to hand her the toothbrush and say 'Clean your teeth'. To be honest, I don't think she understood what I meant and this upset me. She would hold the toothbrush upside down and start cleaning the sink with it. I now help put it in her hand and hold her hand while I mime the action. Sometimes I just clean my own teeth at the same time. It takes my mind off what she cannot do, which breaks my heart and brings a bit of fun into the bathroom when I pull silly faces!"

– Jackie

Again, clean your teeth at the same time to demonstrate what you want them to do. Regular visits to the dentist are important, as your partner may have lost weight, resulting in poorly fitting dentures (if they wear them). When changing their toothbrush, replace it with one that looks the same, as keeping everything consistent helps, although it may be worth trying an electric toothbrush. Cleaning teeth involves a number of stages: taking the cap off the toothpaste, squeezing it and judging the amount onto the toothbrush, putting the toothbrush to the mouth and gently brushing the teeth, turning the water on and knowing to spit out the paste. Remember, their short-term memory loss may make them forget one part of the sequence or they may not recognise the toothbrush. Demonstration can help. Be aware that they may not like the taste of the toothpaste and so an alternative one may need to be tried.

If they enjoy a visit to the hairdresser/barber, continue this, making sure you have plenty of time to get ready to go.

"Barbara still loves a trip to the hairdressers: she's gone to Gina's for over 20 years. She knows her well and actually it was Gina who first noticed changes in her speech. The staff in the salon are very caring and make her feel good, always providing a cup of tea, made to her taste every time. Sometimes I have difficulty getting her there, but I keep some of her shampoo and perfume close at hand to remind her. I open up the bottles and she smells them, and then I say 'Come on then, let's go', and then she usually realises where we're going."

— Tom

Regular hairdressers/barbers can be a great help, as they will have built up a relationship with your partner over time, and they may know their client well. If not, try to find a care-based hairdresser in your area where the staff are trained. If you find it difficult to persuade your partner to go to the hairdresser/barber, they may not be able to understand where you want to take them, as they may not understand the words you are saying. Show them visual prompts to help, such as a photograph of the hairdresser, the logo of the salon, or props such as combs, brushes and rollers. Try using sensory prompts such as shampoos, hairspray or hair cream/wax that they may associate with the salon. If this isn't practical, ask if the hairdressers provide a home visiting service. When you need to care for your partner's hair at home, try to create a bit of a salon atmosphere. Avoid splashing water in their faces and buy brands that don't sting.

Dry shampoos may be an occasional option if you find yourself struggling. Again, keep your partner involved as much as possible. For grooming, a large-handled brush may be better for them to grip. You may find it will help if you have a female member of the family or friend to help with rollers or styling and ask a male family member or friend to help with shaving for men.

When helping with dressing, if your partner has a preference for certain clothes, try to buy a few of the same garment. Put them out in the same place every day such as on the bed, giving choice where possible. When giving them a choice make it between one or two garments and put matching clothes together. Be aware that if the clothes and the bedding are patterned, they may have difficulty recognising them, so it may be better to lay the clothes out on a chair in the order that they need to go on. Again, dressing is made up of a number of stages, break it down into smaller tasks. If one side of their body is more stiff, weak or in pain, help by putting the affected side into the clothes first. When helping them undress, take the unaffected limb out first. Try to opt for looser fitting clothes, bearing in mind that poppers are easier to use than buttons. Velcro can also be a good alternative to buttons and shoelaces. Make sure that shoes and slippers fit well to prevent the risk of falling. Try dancing gently together to make it less threatening and a more pleasurable act. When finished dressing, take the dirty clothing away to avoid them being worn again the next day.

DEMENTIA AND THE TOILET!

The term for being able to control the bladder and bowel is known as continence. Going to the toilet involves a series of complex stages that require memory, dexterity and mobility. A person living with dementia may have difficulties with staying continent for many reasons. They may:

- Lose the sensation that they need to go to the toilet
- Be depressed and lack motivation
- Forget where the toilet is
- Not recognise the toilet due to visual problems
- Have difficulty expressing the need to go, due to speech difficulties
- Have difficulty understanding prompts from loved ones and caregivers
- Struggle with their clothing or may not get to the toilet in time
- Experience changes in diet and drinking
- Not recognise when food has "gone off" which may lead to diarrhoea/food poisoning
- Their medication may be contributing to the incontinence

The first thing I want you to realise is, that this may not be a normal part of the condition, as other physical conditions and medication may also affect a person's ability to stay continent. I know caregivers often don't tend to seek help as they feel embarrassed and conscious of keeping their loved one's dignity. But it is important to speak to your doctor and ask for a continence assessment for them. This is usually done by a specialist continence nurse who will be able to explore the cause in more detail, offer support and advice that may help and thereby reduce the embarrassment and stigma associated with it. An assessment may also include recommending aids such as raised toilet seats and grab rails that will help if your loved one is struggling with mobility.

Things you can do to help include many of the suggestions in this book. This includes making sure there is plenty of light in the home (but avoiding shadows) and that the toilet seat is a contrasting tone from the floor and walls, to help your loved one see more clearly. The recommended lighting level is 300 lux. Be aware that if the colour of the flooring between the outside and the toilet is different or too contrasting, your loved one may see it as a step or a hole. Keep the toilet door open so that it is visible or put a picture sign on the door to identify where the toilet is (making sure the sign is at a height they can see and is not shiny). Encouraging regular trips to the toilet can be an effective way of preventing "accidents". If your loved one becomes a bit resistant to your prompts you could try and say something like "I think I need to go to the toilet before we go out, why don't you go first". Make sure they are eating and drinking well but give their last drink two hours before bedtime to try and prevent continence problems at night.

You may also need to consider using mattress protectors and large absorbent sheets where your partner may be incontinent. This will help them feel more comfortable while giving you less work. Speak to your doctor as there may be a local linen cleaning service in your area. You may also want to put absorbent sheets on any seats that they sit in at home and consider pads (as long as they are changed regularly to avoid their skin from becoming sore and avoid the risk of infection). Here, you will have to be sensitive to their feelings and help your partner realise that it may be comfortable for them to wear pads or specially made undergarments that are absorbent.

Assisting with personal care can help towards your partner's wellbeing, their sense of who they are and their self-esteem. It can also bring you a sense of love and satisfaction when all goes well. However, depending on your relationship and the nature of your relationship, personal care can be challenging to carry out. It needs to be carried out with sensitivity and patience.

"A good friend of our family struggled to help his wife when she flat out refused to bathe or wash her hair......... but he was so patient and kind and regardless, he took her everywhere – greasy hair, wrinkly clothing and all. He walked proudly with her – I have never seen such love in action in all my life. I believe he convinced her to be bathed by a community nurse in the end."

– Carole

Don't be afraid to ask for help if you are finding this difficult. Sometimes a person may prefer a caregiver (not associated with the family) to help them, rather than a close relative.

Don't forget that while you are caring together, humour, music and movement can really help relieve tension, improve the energy in the room and help you keep a deep connection together while you get on with the practical tasks of washing and dressing. I hope that by adopting some of these approaches you will feel a little less stressed and your partner may feel more content and open to receiving your help.

SUMMARY OF CHAPTER EIGHT

How dementia affects appearance and dignity

- Can affect motivation and create apathy
- They may feel embarrassed by loss of control
- Your partner can forget to wash or how to dress, or miss out a stage in the sequence of washing and dressing
- May feel depressed and lack interest in appearance
- Be unable to recognise objects associated with washing and dressing
- May perceive bath mats as holes and/or not recognise the edge of the bath
- May wish to wear the same clothes every day

Approaches to help maintain appearance and dignity

- Take time, don't rush
- Make the bathroom environment relaxing
- Try music in the bedroom
- Let them do as much as possible themselves
- Give prompts and some choice
- Explain what you want them to do, use mime where needed

- Encourage
- Use familiar and favourite products
- Buy a few of the same clothes so you have a clean supply of favourite items
- Keep a rummage box in the bathroom
- Continue with usual hairdresser/barber
- Ask for help

NOTES

Write down your partner's preferences here and what helps and what may create challenges.

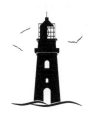

CHAPTER NINE

Understanding Changes in Mood and Behaviour

How to listen and respond to the emotions behind mood and behaviour

When people struggle with getting their point across, are ignored or fearful, the language of emotions steps in.

JANE MULLINS

You may find that your partner's responses, reactions and behaviour changes over time. This can be puzzling and at times upsetting, since their actions may be completely out of character. It can be due to a number of reasons that include not being able to recognise their own needs, being unable to communicate their needs effectively and changes in their ability to reason or make judgements. It is important to remember that their emotions may be driving this and if they don't feel listened to or feel disoriented, they may justifiably become distressed, frustrated and scared.

"Jack used to be such a mild-mannered, loving man, but it seemed like overnight he started to get impatient and sometimes angry. I was frightened: I didn't know what was happening to him. When he was diagnosed with vascular dementia, the doctor told us that it was the disease that was doing this. I was heartbroken but a bit relieved too, as I knew my lovely Jack wouldn't shout at me normally. I now realise he was probably scared. I now take my time and not argue with him when he is adamant about something. He sometimes paces around the room and I take this as a cue to go out. I think he feels a bit trapped sometimes and so do I. My son is good with him: they will go out for a walk together or into his shed, where they putter together on some woodwork or project he used to work on. When he's calmed down, he can speak more easily and let us know what he wants. Sometimes just a change of scenery helps. I think I wind him up but I'm learning to spot what sets him off."

– Margaret

If you can understand why your partner may start acting out of character, you may be able to reassure them and help them to feel more settled. It is worth standing back and trying to work out what is happening in order to help them and yourself in the meantime. If their behaviour alters rapidly, becoming more confused and distressed in a short period of time, it may be caused by a physical problem such as an infection or pain. Does their body language show this, such as grimacing and holding themselves in a certain way? Ask yourself when they last ate or drank, as low blood sugar and dehydration can cause confusion. Your partner may also have other physical conditions that can have an impact on their dementia. Contact your doctor in these instances, as he or she may be able to assess whether there are physical causes to your partner's changes in mood and attitude and treat them effectively.

Try to walk in your partner's shoes. The behaviour is not them; it is because of the dementia and they may be feeling frightened, ignored or frustrated. Difficulties often occur when their needs are not recognised and they may not be able to communicate them to anyone or understand what is being said to them.

"It is it, it is me, I am still me.................... somewhere"

– Malcolm

There may be times when your partner may start to feel anxious when you are out of their sight and they may follow you everywhere you go. It is possible that they feel insecure without you. This is why, I have mentioned in the previous chapters to involve family and friends, so that they don't become solely dependent on you. If this is the case, when you leave the room, explain to them where you are going, maybe it is to the shower or to prepare food. They may retain this knowledge for long enough to give you some time. Try leaving a prop with them that may help keep them interested, for instance a jigsaw, button box, a rummage box (see chapters three and four), whatever works for you. This will differ with everybody but it may give you some valuable moments to yourself. Failing that, try and arrange for friends or family members to visit at these times.

People who have dementia may also experience depression or low mood, which can affect how they respond. This can be caused by the changes in the brain and/or the effects that the dementia has on your partner. It is important to speak with your doctor, as often depression can be masked by the dementia and make the condition appear worse than it is. By following some of the ideas in the previous chapters, you may be able to help their mood and yours. These include:

- Involving family, friends, befrienders and social groups
- Getting out and about in nature
- Bringing light into the home
- Keeping to a routine
- Listening to and validating their feelings
- Sharing food
- Being together, listening to music
- Going through meaningful photographs and objects
- Avoiding challenging and disagreeing with them

Sometimes your partner may become agitated, start pacing or be difficult to placate. If you are concerned and feel out of your depth, try to stand back and ask yourself a few questions, such as:

- Do I see any pattern to this behaviour?
- Is this behaviour in response to certain people?
- When does this behaviour occur?
- Where does this behaviour occur?
- Are they being ignored?
- Has something happened that might have triggered a change in behaviour?

Respond, don't react.......

Try to stay calm, practice some deep slow breathing, and avoid reacting suddenly; show them that you are listening. If something is clearly annoying them, take time to try to find out what it might be (it may be that they need to go to the toilet and they cannot find where to go) and then you are on the way to helping them. We have to try to imagine how we would feel if we felt confused and couldn't communicate our needs.

One day in the Memory Clinic, a lady and her husband were sitting in the waiting room. She was obviously concerned about something and kept standing up and pacing the floor. Her restlessness was turning more to distress and agitation as her husband, who was shattered, tried to get her to sit down many times. She would open and close her bag, clearly looking for something, and play repetitively with her hair. Her husband had a difficult time getting her to come to the clinic and I think he was struggling to cope that morning. I went to sit with them both and realised (as I had fresh eyes and hadn't been awake all night) that she wanted to brush her hair and feel tidy for her appointment now that she knew where she was. Her appearance was very important to her and when she arrived at the clinic she realised that she needed to look presentable. I escorted her to the ladies' room: she brushed her hair and put on her lipstick, and then returned to the waiting room, where she settled and sat down calmly next to him.

I can't begin to understand how exhausting it can be when you are caring for someone living with dementia, but I hope that some of these ideas will help you to understand and maintain a connection with them. I also cannot stress enough, the need to involve other people, as a short break can recharge your batteries and help you to cope better. If you have no family or friends nearby, there may be a befriending service that may be able to offer some help. Contact your local dementia charity or speak to your doctor.

Often people who have dementia display repetitive actions. This can be due to a number of factors, such as not being able to retain information or their needs being misread or ignored. If you have an event planned or a pending appointment, it may be best to avoid telling your partner until much closer to the time. The anticipation of an event may become stuck in their mind, where they are unable to process times and dates. This may make them anxious and cause repetitive questions and habits, as they may retain an awareness that a visit somewhere may be imminent but not able to remember what, where or when. But also, don't spring an appointment on them at the last minute either; you will need to judge when is the best time to let them know they are going out. The use of visual clues to indicate where you will be going may help. Use of clocks and notes around the house may help with their difficulty in judging time.

People who have dementia may also start to walk or pace around, which can be due to a number of factors such as boredom, looking for someone or thinking they should be elsewhere, being in pain, needing the toilet or they may be constipated. Here you need to work out what is the cause and consider a balance between their safety and giving them some freedom. For instance, if your partner becomes adamant about returning home or starts to pace (when you are already at home), they may be thinking of their past home–possibly where they grew up. Sometimes they may be looking for their mother or father. This can be very upsetting for you, but to try to understand that they may be searching for comfort, or they may be feeling lost and worrying that they have a role to play, such as looking after children or going to work.

"I couldn't believe it one morning Marjorie kept pacing up and down and I couldn't settle her. She kept saying that she had to go to work. You could have knocked me over with a feather – she didn't remember she had retired twenty years ago (she was a nurse). I felt so sad. I used to try and reason with her, to tell her that she had retired, but she was adamant that it was time to go on shift. In the end, I took her out in the car for a run and slowly she took notice of other things. We went and had an ice cream by the sea. This seemed to help. I feel deceitful sometimes trying to distract her but she gets so upset otherwise. Telling her she is wrong just makes her feel worse. I suppose I would feel the same."

– Paul

Remember, avoid challenging and confronting. Go with the flow and try to hear the emotion behind your partner's responses and reactions. If they say they are looking for their mother, face them, gain eye contact, put your arm gently on their shoulder and say to them "tell me about her, what was she like?" or something like "yes, she was a wonderful cook, remember her cakes?". That way you are working with their emotions and helping them move into a place of joy while showing them care and love.

It might be better to say "let's go here" instead of "don't go there". Bring out the sensory lifestory and go through some photographs and sensory prompts from the rummage boxes. They may be bored and need some stimulation or gentle exercise. If they were always active in the past, they may be feeling restless now, needing some physical movement.

"One of the ladies who lived in the care home always felt the need to go outside as dusk set in and would become quite agitated if she thought that she couldn't go. After speaking with her son, we found out that she had always fed her chickens at that time and shut them in their coop to stop the fox from attacking them. So, every evening one of our staff would accompany her out into the garden and they would both return having had a lovely chat and a walk, ready to return inside for bed. It didn't matter that there weren't any chickens, we helped her continue her lifelong habit that she associated with dusk and she was happy."

– Rita, Care Home Nurse Manager

Look for some items around the house that may engage your partner in activities, helping them to focus on where they are at the time. For instance, if your partner worked in an office, find an old typewriter and desk and create an office space in the corner of your living room. Create a meaningful distraction from their distress that responds to their needs. This doesn't have to be mentally taxing. Perhaps something to keep them interested or engaged, such as the use of a button box to rummage through or something associated with their background (this could include folding clothes, sharpening pencils or feeling books, seed packets, pieces of wood and sandpaper– whatever you think they might sense a meaningful association with). This doesn't always have to involve objects that your partner associates with from the past; tastes in music, interests and food preferences can change, so you may need to be creative in your thinking.

One gentleman I cared for was a retired university professor who felt content when given a basket of socks to match and put together. Sorting through buttons, materials etc. can give a feeling of a sense of purpose and occupation.

It is hard for us to move away from seeing our partner as the person they were before they had dementia in terms of their previous ability, as we are often defined by our roles and jobs in life. But if you can understand what is happening in the present moment and keep an open mind to what keeps them content, you can learn to connect together and help them to feel calmer.

I know of a care home where a number of the residents wandered and insisted on leaving the Home, becoming agitated when not able to leave through the front door. The Manager realised that they had all spent their whole adult lives getting up and going out to work. Instead of contradicting them and stopping them, the staff put a bus stop in the grounds of the Home. Here the residents would wander outside and stand together chatting while waiting for the bus. When it didn't turn up, they had all naturally distracted themselves from the urgent feeling of needing to get to work, and clearly enjoyed a sociable time together before returning back into the Home for a drink and snack.

It is difficult sometimes because you may feel that you are being deceitful. But you need to realise that by being creative in your responses your goal is to keep you and your partner feeling safe and-contented. As previously mentioned your partner may be less likely to pace around if they are engaged in some activity, make sure they are not hungry, thirsty or in pain and help them to the toilet. If they become frustrated when they arrive at a dead end, you may help by putting a chair nearby and a box of objects to fiddle with or a familiar picture; something to engage and interest them.

If your partner is still independent and goes out alone, you may be concerned about them getting lost, or if they have a tendency to wander, you may wish to consider using a GPS watch or phone that can track their whereabouts. There are ethical concerns regarding tracking, as your partner may feel that they are under constant surveillance, however, in my view, it would give peace of mind if, as the dementia progresses they are at a real risk of getting lost. It is also worth putting a medic alert card and contact details of family and friends (and car licence plate numbers, if they are still driving) on business sized cards in their bag or wallet. An engraved bracelet/watch that gives their name and contact details alongside a statement explaining their condition is also helpful. Part of the difficulty of caring for someone who has dementia involves helping them to stay independent for as long as possible while making sure that they are safe. Making sure you have friends and family to support you in this helps you to feel that you are not alone when having to make decisions. If you have no family or friends to help, get in touch with your local dementia charity, café or groups such as singing, they will welcome you and you will feel more supported.

Some types of dementia can impact on the person's social graces, where they may curse and swear, become euphoric or express themselves in sexually inappropriate ways. This doesn't always happen but if it does, remember, again, it is the dementia speaking and acting and not your partner. Speak to family and friends and explain to them that the damage in their brain causes your partner to respond in this way. Try and identify any triggers which may set this off with a view to preventing it. Such as keeping their hands occupied with activities and sensory objects as suggested in previous chapters. You may find it useful to fill out the behaviour journal at the end of this chapter. For instance, you may notice that they tend to lift their clothes, this could be because they need the toilet and do not recognise the sensation. Certainly, if their social graces deteriorate even further I would recommend that you speak with your doctor.

I hope that by reading this chapter you will have come to understand that your partner's dementia may cause them to respond in ways that are out of character and that it is not intentional. By adopting some of the approaches suggested you may be able to minimise the indignity and embarrassment for you both while trying to stay re-connected together.

SUMMARY OF CHAPTER NINE

How dementia affects responses, reactions and behaviour

- Being unable to communicate needs
- Being unable to recognise own needs
- Changes in ability to judge, assess risk and reason
- Disorientation to time and place
- Fear, loss of control

Approaches to help with maintaining wellbeing

- All points in previous chapters will help
- Stay calm and show that you are listening
- Avoid challenging and being confrontational
- Look for triggers, use the behaviour diary
- Be aware they may need the toilet or may be in pain
- Be aware of the environment, keep it light and clutter free
- Contact doctor if behaviour changes suddenly as this may be due to other physical factors
- Consider assistive technology to help with disorientation

NOTES

Date: Comment:

NOTES

Date:	Comment:

NOTES

Date: **Comment:**

NOTES

Date: Comment:

Date & time of day	
Where	
Who was present?	
How did your partner respond?	
What was happening (triggers) e.g. think of sights, sounds, smells, light/dark, weather?	
Write down strategies that have helped minimise your partner's changing responses, reactions and behaviour.	

It might be helpful to note down what was happening at the time that your partner's behaviour changed. You may see a pattern and find ways of avoiding the triggers which in turn could help them stay contented. This will be helpful information when speaking with your doctor.

Date & time of day	
Where	
Who was present?	
How did your partner respond?	
What was happening (triggers) e.g. think of sights, sounds, smells, light/ dark, weather?	
Write down strategies that have helped minimise your partner's changing responses, reactions and behaviour.	

Date & time of day	
Where	
Who was present?	
How did your partner respond?	
What was happening (triggers) e.g. think of sights, sounds, smells, light/ dark, weather?	
Write down strategies that have helped minimise your partner's changing responses, reactions and behaviour.	

Date & time of day	
Where	
Who was present?	
How did your partner respond?	
What was happening (triggers) e.g. think of sights, sounds, smells, light/ dark, weather?	
Write down strategies that have helped minimise your partner's changing responses, reactions and behaviour.	

Date & time of day	
Where	
Who was present?	
How did your partner respond?	
What was happening (triggers) e.g. think of sights, sounds, smells, light/ dark, weather?	
Write down strategies that have helped minimise your partner's changing responses, reactions and behaviour.	

Date & time of day	
Where	
Who was present?	
How did your partner respond?	
What was happening (triggers) e.g. think of sights, sounds, smells, light/dark, weather?	
Write down strategies that have helped minimise your partner's changing responses, reactions and behaviour.	

Date & time of day	
Where	
Who was present?	
How did your partner respond?	
What was happening (triggers) e.g. think of sights, sounds, smells, light/dark, weather?	
Write down strategies that have helped minimise your partner's changing responses, reactions and behaviour.	

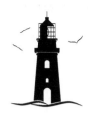

CHAPTER TEN

Altered States: Hallucinations, Delusions, Misperceptions

Try new approaches to avoid distress

Life is a balance between holding on and letting go.

RUMI

Sometimes dementia can cause a person to experience a different reality to our own. This may include seeing, hearing, tasting or smelling something that isn't present (hallucinations). Also, perhaps, the inability to recognise objects, people, tastes or sounds (misperceptions) and/or having a fixed belief that is not true (delusions). Strong feelings are often attached to that reality and it is important to acknowledge those feelings.

"I got so frightened – he started shouting at the TV. I know he used to shout at the news sometimes before, but this was different. I turned the TV off and he kept shouting at something and saying there were elephants coming through the window. He went out into the street and was telling our neighbours to get rid of them. None of us knew what to do but I just found myself going along with him. I called my son and he came over and gradually he calmed him down and we went back into the house. I rang the doctor who came and offered some advice. They don't always want to prescribe drugs, and they told me that they could make the dementia worse. I don't put the TV on anymore, as that would seem to trigger his mood. We listen to music instead. It is hard, as I like to watch the news, so I wait until he goes out with my son and then put my feet up, ignore the housework and catch up on what's been happening in the outside world."

– Laura

Hallucinations are more common in Lewy Body Dementia (LBD) and Parkinson's disease dementia (although they can occur in Alzheimer's disease and other types of dementia). They may include seeing animals or people that aren't there. It may happen only occasionally or more frequently, sometimes daily. Your partner's reality is different to your own at this moment in time and they will have a fixed belief that what they are experiencing is real.

"What they are able to imagine becomes more real to them."

– Dr Oliver Sacks

This is usually caused by damage to the area of the brain affected by the dementia and/or changes in the neurochemicals in the brain. Sometimes characters from television may appear very real and in the room with them. It may be difficult for your partner to work out what is actual and what is virtual from televisions and screens. This may or may not frighten them, but if it does, I would suggest turning off the television and reducing the sensory overload (voices from the radio may also apply here).

If they appear to be experiencing hallucinations, then the first thing to do is to ask yourself:

- Are they upset by this?
- Is their behaviour being affected?
- Are they at risk?
- Are they frightened?

Use the journal at the end of this chapter to see if you can identify the triggers. Sometimes, people may not be concerned by their hallucinations, but if they are, here are some tips to help.

Don't attempt to challenge your partner or reason with them, as what they are experiencing is real to them. They are more likely to become upset and agitated if they feel that nobody believes them.

Try to find a distraction. Sometimes hallucinations may occur in specific settings: if possible, move to another room, go out for a walk, or maybe listen to some gentle music. Be mindful that certain smells may be a trigger. It may be worth getting your partner involved in some activities to help distract them. It is often trial and error, and you will get to know what they enjoy doing and what may help. Monitor for triggers, such as:

- Time of day
- What they were doing just before the hallucinations/delusions occurred?
- Where they were at the time?
- How long did it last?

What may seem to be a hallucination may possibly be more of a misperception, such as mistaking one object for another or mistaking who they believe they are seeing. Sometimes your partner may not recognise their older self in the mirror and this can be quite frightening. If a reflection in a mirror causes distress, cover the mirror or get someone to help you attach a blind to it, so that you are still able to use it but it is not visible to them. If they have poor eyesight, make sure they have regular appointments with an optician (and hearing tests) as the changes in the brain may affect what they are sensing. Suggest moving into a different room, de-clutter the space and change the lighting, as sometimes shadows, dark rooms and patterns can cause misperceptions.

Sometimes your partner may communicate an idea that is false, which may appear bizarre and they might become paranoid, such as believing that family members are stealing from them. This is a fixed belief and can be very upsetting for family members and friends. Think about the emotion behind this; it may be due to fear, feeling insecure and frustration at losing control. Try not to take this personally and avoid challenging the belief or trying to reason with them, because what they feel is their reality. Don't forget it is the dementia speaking. You may try to dispel their belief by saying, "I meant to tell you that I popped your money in the bank" and show them some correspondence. Once again, validate their feelings, I would try to sit down with them, show that you are listening and you could write a list of what they think they are missing. Chances are, the immediate emotion is dispelled and by offering reassurance, your partner may become distracted from their belief. If they accuse you of taking or hiding something, try saying "I think I saw it in the other room" and take them in there to look. If you keep small rummage boxes of interesting objects in each room (without being cluttered), they may become pleasantly distracted.

People can be mistaken for other members in the family, such as a son being seen as his father. There may be times when you may want to try to bring your partner back to your reality and sometimes, earlier on in the condition, this may be possible. But it is important not to confront or contradict them. As the condition progresses, it may be better to let it go and not correct them. Try to stay in the moment: your partner needs to feel that they are safe and cared for. This can be extremely upsetting for you but try to follow these approaches and you may feel a little more in control and manage to dispel your partner's distress. As mentioned before, this may not happen to your partner, but if it does you now have some approaches to follow that may help.

Have you thought of a creating a dementia first aid kit? You could gather together a small number of meaningful objects such as keys, watch, loose change, a handkerchief that may be touched, smelt and seen, some lavender or pleasant scents which may help bring your partner back into a calmer state. If you make it small enough, you could carry it with you to help when away from home. It could be a mini version of their lifestory that involves a sensory distraction from their upset.

If you struggle with this, I would suggest talking to your doctor about counselling and support to help you and ask them to recommend a local support group. As I have stressed throughout this book, try to maintain contact with family and friends, knowing that isolation from others is unhealthy. If you are getting good support, you are in a better position to care.

If hallucinations and/or delusions continue over time or if they involve a number of senses all at once, it is important that you consult your doctor, as they may also be caused by other physical complaints such as infection, pain or even the side effects of some medication. Let your doctor know if there are any triggers (use the diary at the back of this chapter), what your partner sensed and how they reacted.

I hope that this chapter has given you more of an idea of why your partner may be showing changes in their behaviour and provide you with some advice and approaches that may help you through the difficult times.

SUMMARY OF CHAPTER TEN

How dementia can affect reality

- May see, hear, taste or smell something that is not present (hallucinations)
- Inability to recognise objects, people, tastes or sounds (misperceptions)
- Experience a fixed belief that is not true (delusions)

Approaches to help dispel distress

- Stay calm and offer reassurance (when required)
- Avoid challenging, contradicting and confronting
- Look for triggers and fill out the journal overleaf
- Turn down radios, televisions and computers
- Keep the room light, avoiding shadows
- Move to a different space
- Involve friends and family
- Practice relaxation and acupressure (see chapter 11)
- Contact your doctor

NOTES

Date: **Comment:**

NOTES

Date: **Comment:**

How did your partner react? e.g. What did they see, hear, say?	
Date & time of day	
Where?	
Who was present?	
What were the triggers e.g. think of sights, sounds, smells, light/ dark, weather?	
How long did it last?	
What helped it to stop?	

(This may not be applicable to you and your partner)

It might be helpful to note down what was happening at the time of your partner's hallucinations, delusions or fixed beliefs. You may see a pattern and find ways of avoiding the triggers which will help them stay contented. This may be helpful information when speaking with your doctor.

How did your partner react? e.g. What did they see, hear, say?	
Date & time of day	
Where?	
Who was present?	
What were the triggers e.g. think of sights, sounds, smells, light/ dark, weather?	
How long did it last?	
What helped it to stop?	

How did your partner react? e.g. What did they see, hear, say?	
Date & time of day	
Where?	
Who was present?	
What were the triggers e.g. think of sights, sounds, smells, light/ dark, weather?	
How long did it last?	
What helped it to stop?	

How did your partner react? e.g. What did they see, hear, say?	
Date & time of day	
Where?	
Who was present?	
What were the triggers e.g. think of sights, sounds, smells, light/ dark, weather?	
How long did it last?	
What helped it to stop?	

How did your partner react? e.g. What did they see, hear, say?	
Date & time of day	
Where?	
Who was present?	
What were the triggers e.g. think of sights, sounds, smells, light/ dark, weather?	
How long did it last?	
What helped it to stop?	

How did your partner react? e.g. What did they see, hear, say?	
Date & time of day	
Where?	
Who was present?	
What were the triggers e.g. think of sights, sounds, smells, light/ dark, weather?	
How long did it last?	
What helped it to stop?	

CHAPTER ELEVEN

Caring for the Caregiver

Quick and easy ways to nurture and replenish yourself

You yourself, as much as anybody in the entire universe, deserve your love and affection.

BUDDHA

I don't need to tell you about the difficulties and challenges you experience when caring for your loved one. Do not ignore the emotional, physical and social upheaval that you are experiencing. Relationships change due to the nature of dementia and the aim of *Finding the Light* is to help support you in this. I cannot stress enough, the importance of caring for yourself in order to be able to care for your partner. If you become stressed, start to struggle and feel isolated, you won't be able to care for them. There is a chance that you are not getting your needs met and at some point, you may feel resentful about this, and guilty for having these feelings. Even with all that I have covered in this book, you may very well be grieving for your partner as the person they were and the losses in life associated with these changes. It is important to recognise this and speak with your doctor. You may find specialist grief counselling a help, or as mentioned in the last chapter, a support group may offer you some comfort. Do not cope alone.

Below are a few ideas that may help you feel better (some have already been discussed throughout the book but they are worth repeating):

Firstly, slow down, stand back and re-connect with who you are–recognise your amazing self. Make sure you speak with others and don't be too proud or embarrassed to ask for help; engage other people in your life to offer support. Don't wait until you are too tired and exhausted, put plans in place now. Often friends and other family members start to move away. Usually this is because they don't know what to do or say, and find it difficult to cope. Get them to read this book, and use your partner's sensory lifestory. Try to create a rota of friends who could pop in just for an hour or could go out with your partner out for a walk on a specific day. Involve them in reminiscence practices such as picnics, going through photographs and props around the home. In the meantime, you need to go out to meet friends, go shopping, to the cinema, whatever you love. It is important to do this and not to feel guilty. By making yourself set plans you will be more likely to continue caring and connecting with your partner for longer and they need to connect with other people too.

By giving yourself an hour, maybe in the morning and possibly the afternoon, you will be able to practice self-care and be in a much better position as a caregiver. Little and often is the way to look after yourself. This time must be spent caring for you. The household chores will have to wait; you will have more energy to do them when you have recharged your batteries. Speak to your doctor and ask what help is available, and contact local support groups, which may be able to offer a befriending service or some day-care activities.

RELAXATION 1

Learn to be in the moment: sit quietly for five to ten minutes and think of a word, prayer or mantra you can focus on. Let the word mean how you would like to feel. You may quietly repeat to yourself words such as Calm, Peace, Bliss, Breathe, Love. Set the alarm so that you do sit for the full time and try to create a special space in the home for you to do this. If your partner won't leave your side, repeat the words gently out loud so they may feel the vibration and sound, which may have a calming effect on them.

I would certainly recommend you try the quick 5-minute relaxation techniques below:

When you have a shower, bath (where possible) or even pop your feet in a foot spa try to use some calming smells such as 5 drops of lavender. Practice your word or mantra and try to love your body and reconnect with yourself. At any time when you feel overwhelmed or stressed, take a deep breath and repeat your chosen word until the feeling fades. As a reminder, write your word or words on post it notes and place them around your house, in the bathroom, on the fridge door, by the front door – keep them everywhere. Often, as caregivers, we can condition ourselves to feeling stressed over time so we now need to re-condition ourselves to feel calmer. With practice, this approach can change the energies in the home from tension to calmness. If you have the space in your home, create one room into a retreat with a comfortable chair, plants and gentle music. If you feel guilty about your thoughts and feelings, embrace the guilt, then let it go – visualise it floating away attached to a balloon. Guilt can be very damaging and does not serve you, let it go. Humour helps – if you can put some comedy on the television or radio, a good laugh can really lift your spirits. Slapstick can be a great example of the power of non-verbal communication and often may help you both re-connect together. Pets can also be a source of comfort to you both.

As mentioned throughout the book, try to rest when your partner does. Even ten minutes of sitting still, closing your eyes, taking slow deep breaths and repeating your word can help recharge the batteries. We can become irritable and find it harder to cope when we don't eat, so make sure that you prepare some quick and easy foods for yourself (see chapter seven). Again, little and often may work better for you. Remind yourself of how remarkable you are. Learn to reflect on the day. It is helpful to reflect on what went well and what didn't. Think back and instead of engaging with guilt, think of how you could change how you approached certain aspects of the day, using this book as a guide. Don't be hard on yourself – it can take time and many attempts to make changes, you are amazing. Write a diary if you can, as getting your thoughts and feelings out onto paper can help you feel better. Then listen to music or if possible find a good book or film to enjoy.

RELAXATION 2

For five minutes in the morning and five minutes at night, send yourself loving kindness messages. Sit in a quiet place, where you will not be disturbed, and turn off all distractions. Close your eyes and say to yourself.......

- I am happy
- I am joyful
- I am blessed

- I am well
- I am loved
- I am valued

Really try to feel what you are saying as research has shown that our brain believes what we tell it! Note how you feel afterwards.

"Our brain is the hard drive and our thoughts are the software"

**– Carole Fawcett, Counsellor &
Clinical Hypnotherapist**

OTHER WAYS OF RELIEVING STRESS

The use of aromatherapy and acupressure can help you return to a calmer state and can be adopted quite easily and over a short period of time. It can also help your partner. Try a hand massage with three drops of Lavender (make sure that the smell doesn't trigger any unwanted emotions). There are also areas on the wrist and ears that, when massaged can help reduce stress.

RELAXATION 3

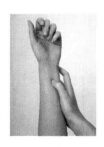

Measure down with three fingers from the wrist to the area shown below. Note where your third finger touches the middle of your wrist and place your thumb on that spot and apply firm pressure until it feels mildly uncomfortable. Apply enough pressure to interrupt the normal blood flow but not so that it causes pain. Hold this point and gently knead your thumb in a tight circular movement for about 2 minutes. Repeat on your other wrist and you will feel much calmer. This point can also help for nausea.

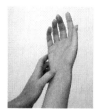

You can also use your thumb to apply a firm pressure at the spot where your wrist forms a crease with your hand for 2 minutes, this can really help relieve any tension you may have.

The ears are also sensitive to massage, use your thumb and forefinger and pull your lobes down gently and massage the inner surface of both ears for 2 minutes. You will feel more soothed all over.

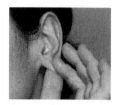

Try and get in the habit of a quick gentle massage throughout the day. If you feel less stressed, your partner may sense your calmness and intuitively mirror you.

I hope this chapter will have shown you the importance of valuing yourself and help you when in the midst of life. By offering you these approaches you may feel better equipped to cope with any difficult times and help you stay well while keeping a deep connection with your partner.

SUMMARY OF CHAPTER ELEVEN

Slow down and stand back.

- Engage the help of others – create a rota of visitors, stress to them that a regular hourly visit would be helpful. Let them read this book, use your loved one's sensory lifestory with them, reminiscence.
- Note your feelings, speak to your doctor about grief counselling or a support group
- Sit and Be for five to ten minutes at a time, slow your breathing and repeat a chosen word, prayer or mantra. Such as: Calm, Peace, Bliss, Breathe, Love.
- Use aromatherapy and massage your acupressure points regularly throughout the day.
- Humour helps – put some comedy on the television or radio, it can lift your spirits.
- Rest and eat when your loved one does – little and often where possible.
- Reflect on the day, using this book to help you change what didn't go well. Reflect on what also went well, more often than not you will think of something.
- Read the main points at the end of each chapter and apply as many as you can, as they aim to help you as well as your partner.

NOTES

_____

_____

_____

_____

_____

_____

_____

_____

_____

_____

_____

_____

_____

_____

_____

_____

_____

_____

_____

_____

Write down things that you like to do that help you relax. You may want to create a relaxation box for yourself which includes essential oils, music and relaxation mantras or sayings.

NOTES

NOTES

NOTES

CHAPTER TWELVE

Considering Care

What to look for in choosing caregivers,
respite and care homes

It's not how much you do, but how much
love you put in the doing.

MOTHER TERESA

This is probably the chapter that you do not wish to read or do not want to face. But it is important to realise that there may come a time when you will need to seek professional help. This may involve a caregiver coming into your home, respite care for you, a hospital admission, or more permanently, finding a care home for your partner. You may just need somebody to act as a companion or befriender for your partner while you go out, or you may need them to be more involved in helping them provide some personal care such as

173

washing and dressing. Whatever your partner's needs are, it is so important that the person providing the help understands the nature of dementia and has had training. Some people are more natural in their approach than others. Speak to your doctor or ask your dementia charity about recommending such services.

"I just needed a break now and again to pop to the shops and meet my friends for a quick coffee. This was getting harder to do. I didn't feel relaxed leaving him at home on his own for more than half an hour. Some of our friends used to call, but that was getting less and less. I knew that Bruce needed some male company and was so pleased to find Matthew through the local dementia caregivers group. He would call every Wednesday morning as planned and sit with Bruce and they would go over old times, talking about football and their first cars! He knew how to help him when he couldn't get his words out and he really turned into a great friend. Once he had gone through his lifestory a couple of times, it was as if he had known Bruce years ago. He was a natural. It made me feel less guilty for having a bit of time to myself, I found myself having something to look forward to again while Bruce had a great time too."

– Angela

This is where your partner's sensory lifestory will be of great help. As it can provide much information to help them understand your partner and all aspects of his/her life when they may be unable to communicate easily. It would also be a good idea to let them read through this book to see your notes after each chapter, which will provide valuable information about what can really help and benefit your partner. (Unless of course you have written very personal accounts that you would rather keep private).

When you start to introduce a befriender or caregiver to your partner they may not feel happy about the "stranger" at first, as they may be unable to make a rational judgement about your decision or your choice of the person. I would recommend that you say that they have come to help you with the household chores as you are getting tired. The befriender/caregiver may need to visit a number of times before you are able to leave them with your partner alone. But gradually your partner should get used to them being around and hopefully they will develop a friendship together. Once they have built up a good relationship, the befriender/caregiver may take your partner out for some fresh air and a gentle walk.

There may be a time when your partner has to go into hospital whether planned or as an emergency. I would recommend always keeping a bag packed with some essentials in a spare cupboard to avoid having to think about what you need to take in order to reduce your stress. Keep a copy of up to date information regarding your partner's background, medication and preferences, to help hospital staff understand their needs (see appendix). This may help save time and give you some breathing space when you may be feeling overwhelmed. Don't forget that your copy of *Finding the Light* will also have some important information that may help hospital staff. Going into hospital can be a very disorientating experience for someone who has dementia, if you can set up a rota of friends and family who know your partner well and can visit, this will help, as hospital staff are often very busy and unable to give your partner the time they need. If you or a friend or family member can be there at mealtimes and any times where you feel they may become stressed, such as early evening, you may be able to help them relax. Make sure they have some familiar comforting objects with them such as their playlist with headphones, comfort blanket and something to keep them occupied. (Remember Suzy's comments in chapter five about her mother's bedside cabinet). If they are still reading, books and magazines can be a great help. Of course, it is always better to try and avoid going into hospital, speak to your doctor about giving necessary treatment at home where your partner will feel comfortable.

There may be times when you are unsure of how long you will be able to carry on caring for your partner. However, it is important to consider involving other caregivers before you reach crisis point. I am hoping that following the advice in this book, may have delayed this somewhat. One option would be respite care, where your partner may stay in residential care for a short time in order for you to have a rest from your caring duties and know that they are being cared for. Consult page 178, as finding a suitable place for respite may be befitting for a more permanent home later on.

As time goes on, I would recommend thinking of a scenario where you feel your partner will need more permanent professional care. This may relate to your own health or your partner's. It may be an event where their safety was compromised, such as walking further away from home or at night, or where your health is being affected. Whatever it is, if you can identify the scenario before it happens, it may make you more prepared for the decision at that time. Speak to your family and friends, you really need to get their support here.

"As your partner's needs change and you start to think about a care home environment, you should never feel any guilt in considering this. It just means that their needs have changed where your health and wellbeing is affected to a point where you may not be at your fittest or best to support them. This means that all your knowledge and experience of caring for them just needs to be addressed in a different way, to protect your partner's and your health and well-being. Good care homes encourage and support the main caregiver to participate in the planning of the care in this new environment and being involved can still be a rewarding experience for you as well as your loved one – just in a different setting."

– Lorraine, Care Home Manager

Before finding a care home, I would recommend speaking with your doctor about a care needs assessment to make sure that the home is able to provide the right level of care for your partner. But in the meantime, you can start to explore what is available locally so that you feel more prepared and in control of the situation. Do not wait for a crisis to happen. The next page offers some advice when choosing a care home.

WHAT TO CONSIDER WHEN CHOOSING A CARE HOME

Drop in to the care home with a view to making an appointment. This way you will see the home, warts and all and help you make a judgement on how the staff communicate with you. You will also get a general feel of the place. The staff will understandably be busy and may not have much time set aside to spend with you, but they should communicate with you well and help you make an appointment. You will probably decide there and then if you actually want to go back.

Look out for recommendations, speak to your local dementia charity, doctor or memory clinic who may be able to give you some feedback. You may wish to look at the most recent inspection report of the home.

Where possible, find a local home in your community, this way your partner may know some of the residents and strike up a friendship and they may feel more connected to the area. Also, it will be easier for your friends to visit.

Check if they allow opportunities for you, your family and friends to take your partner out.

Follow your gut instinct. We are usually right, as when something doesn't feel right, then it probably isn't. But if you feel an instant warmth to the place that is usually a good sign. Remember your emotions are going to be all over the place. I would recommend you always take someone with you.

Is the environment bright? Think back to chapter five and how important light, clutter free and lovely views are. Is there a secure garden? Are the residents able to sit outside? If there is more than one door out into the garden that can be great for those who like to walk, as they may be free to saunter in and out as they please.

Do the residents look happy? there may of course be some who may experience some stress, so it would be advisable to visit a few times before you make the decision as you may have caught someone in a difficult moment. The important thing to note is how the staff respond.

Do the residents look stimulated and interested?

Are they respectfully dressed and well groomed?

Is the manager responsive to your questions and helpful?

Do they provide person centred care?

Are the staff respectful of the residents?

Are the staff trained in dementia care?

Would your partner have a named member of staff responsible for their care?

Are there areas provided that encourage socialising? Some homes have dedicated reminiscence rooms that help the residents feel more at home.

Is the home mindful if your partner has young onset dementia? You do not want your partner to feel isolated. Do they respect your partner's interests and plan to incorporate them into his/her day? Take some time to stop and listen, are the sounds of the home pleasant? Is the background atmosphere pleasing? Do they provide a programme of individualised activities? Are they interested in your partner's sensory lifestory that will help with their care planning? Can you visit at any time and have meals with your partner? The home should do all they can to make the transition a gentle one that includes your involvement.

Would your partner be able to bring in some furniture for their room, so they feel a sense of familiarity?

Are special diets provided if required? Ask to see the menu, is there a choice of meals?

Where residents become unwell, will they see a local doctor? Do they have access to other services such as chiropody, counselling, opticians and dentists? Is there a call system for a person requiring help?

Do they have measures in place to reduce the risk of falls?

Do they arrange organised trips and partake in special celebrations?

Do they have regular exercise and fresh air? Are they accommodating and respectful of cultural differences?

This is by no means an exhaustive list and you may want to consider asking more questions that are specific to your partner's needs.

Once you have made the decision I would recommend that you ask for some legal help to look over the contract before you sign, just to make sure you are protected. Do not underestimate the stress that you may be under at this moment in time and having someone else cast their eyes over it will give you some extra support. The contract should cover the cost of care and the notice period of any price increases, alongside any required advance payments. Make sure it covers the type of accommodation and the level of care your partner will be requiring, alongside any additional costs such as laundry, hairdressing and chiropody.

When planning your partner's possible move into permanent residential care, it is worth considering a period of transition. I would firstly recommend visiting the home a few times together and enjoy an afternoon tea there (this would also be a good idea before planning respite care), so that it becomes a familiar place and is associated with pleasant memories. Take your partner's lifestory with you to introduce to the staff, making sure that their current likes and dislikes are written down (such as food and drink preferences, hobbies, music, how they communicate best). It may be worth taking *Finding the Light* with you and going through your most current notes at the end of each chapter with the staff. They will also get the chance to know you both as a couple. On the day of the move, ask a key family member or friend to be at the home to greet you and your partner when you arrive. This also helps towards making your partner feel secure by creating a sense of familiarity. Create a rota of family members and friends who can be on hand to help for the next few weeks, popping in to visit each day, which will take the pressure off you while you choose when to visit and take care of yourself at this time. Try and get them to introduce your partner's lifestory to the staff so that they continue to connect with your partner in meaningful ways and provide familiar activities around them.

As you can see, there is much to consider and this can feel like a very daunting time. Don't underestimate how you will be feeling, be kind to yourself, make sure close family and friends are there to support you. This will be a very sad time where you will be feeling a sense of loss and grief. If you haven't already, ask your doctor to refer you for counselling or support. It is important that you allow yourself to grieve and be gentle with yourself. Don't forget the advice in chapter eleven; that is still helpful for you now. But also, try and remember that your connection to your partner isn't lost, you may find that you can spend more quality time with them now and may enjoy each other's company more; quality of time not quantity of time.

Many people who have dementia can feel more settled when they are with other people living with the condition as there is less pressure to communicate verbally and act on a cognitive level. The care home should offer individualised activities based on your partner's lifestory that you should be able to also participate in, where you can be fully in the moment with them. You will have more energy and time to spend with your partner in a meaningful way whilst knowing that they are having 24-hour care and companionship.

"After four nights on the trot of her wandering at night, I had no sleep. I started to feel irate and shouted at her. I was so exhausted. I lost all feelings for Marjorie and for myself. I felt hopeless, I couldn't take care of her properly anymore and she looked unkempt. Not like the beautiful well turned out lady I had married. When I caught sight of myself in the mirror, I didn't even recognise who I was, as I hadn't had a shave in days and didn't recognise what I had become. I never thought this day would come, well I think I'd blocked it out. If you don't think about it, it won't happen!! I spoke to Jackie, our 'singing for fun' organiser who was very supportive and told me that it was totally normal to feel like this and that we had to consider a care home for Marjorie. That night I cried so much, but looking back I think some of it was out of relief as well as despair. Jackie stayed with Marjorie while my daughter came around to visit some care homes with me. It is the hardest thing I have ever done in my life. But since she has been in the home we have both spent some lovely times together again. I pretend that I am dating her again, (even though I don't think she always knows I am her husband). I can still take her to our singing group, the difference now is that she looks well turned out and so do I!! Then we go back and have lunch together at the home. I get my rest and we still have a lovely time together. There are times when I think I should have done this sooner and not struggled on for both our sakes."

– Tom

Don't forget that all that you have learned throughout this book has helped you care for your partner living with a very complex condition. You will have learned and continue to find valuable ways to communicate with them as they have struggled to get their point across, each time strengthening your connection together. You will have understood the power of using the senses as you continue to reminisce about the past together. This will also be the key to getting others to communicate with your partner in a meaningful way and will greatly help the caregiving staff. You will have created your own lifestory too that will help you value your life together as you were before the dementia and while living through the condition at all stages.

By understanding how the dementia has affected them, you have learned to and will continue to walk side by side with them, making gentle positive changes to your environment as you have gone along. You have understood how to nurture them and yourself with food and drink and learned how to help them and you relax together and when apart. You will have so much to share with the professional caregivers and the notes you have written in this book will help that transition for both you and your partner. If you have followed the tips and advice throughout *Finding the Light* I hope you will remain connected together in a way possibly never expected. I wish you well.

NOTES

Write down specific questions to ask and any comments you wish to make when considering professional care. This may include points made when meeting potential befrienders or caregivers or when visiting a residential care home.

NOTES

NOTES

NOTES

NOTES

NOTES

Date:

Question:

Answer:

Date:

Question:

Answer:

Use these pages to write down any questions you wish to ask your doctor, health professional and/or legal representative and write down their responses.

QUESTION SHEET

Date:

Question:

Answer:

Date:

Question:

Answer:

Date:

Question:

Answer:

Date:

Question:

Answer:

Date:

Question:

Answer:

Date:

Question:

Answer:

QUESTION SHEET

Date:

Question:

Answer:

Date:

Question:

Answer:

Date:

Question:

Answer:

Date:

Question:

Answer:

Date:

Question:

Answer:

Date:

Question:

Answer:

QUESTION SHEET

Date:

Question:

Answer:

Date:

Question:

Answer:

Date:

Question:

Answer:

QUESTION SHEET

Date:

Question:

Answer:

Date:

Question:

Answer:

Date:

Question:

Answer:

QUESTION SHEET

Date:

Question:

Answer:

Date:

Question:

Answer:

Date:

Question:

Answer:

Epilogue

By reading *Finding the Light* you will see that the ethos is a spiritual one. When I speak of spiritual, I mean in the sense of one's life having meaning and purpose. *Finding the Light* offers hope and strength to all those affected by dementia; whether you have the diagnosis yourself or are living or caring for someone who has been diagnosed with the condition.

Finding the Light brings out the love, trust and creativity of relationships with a belief and a faith in self. By recognising both your needs, you can move towards healing. When I speak of healing, I do not mean curing–these are two very different things. By connecting the human spirit to each other, you can continue to live a meaningful life together, whether living alone, in the same home or if your loved one is in residential care.

Ways of connecting include being in touch with nature, whether it is walking outdoors, or, if not practical, asking your friends and families to bring nature indoors to you. Don't forget how important your senses are–small plants, flowers, shells, and the sound of birdsong all help us to feel alive and connected to something greater. If you have grandchildren or young children, encourage them to bring in something seasonal such as conkers, blackberries and strawberries.

Whilst in the midst of caring, we tend to forget to look for the positive aspects to life; it is important for your sense of wellbeing to find something that you are grateful for—there will be something, look for the magic moments in the day, however, small they may feel.

The use of music is powerful in lifting moods: if you find yourself having a "down" day, put on some uplifting music, and connect with others, as it can and frequently does help.

Appendix

Hospital Admission Kit

Your partner:

- 2 changes of familiar clothing (labelled) including underwear
- Nightwear and slippers
- A toilet bag with soap, flannel, toothbrush, toothpaste, shampoo and hand wipes, Lavender (if appropriate)
- Photographs and meaningful objects that may provide comfort
- Music player and headphones with their playlist
- Wallet or purse with a little money
- Any medication or treatment that your partner takes regularly or as required
- A bag for clothes (to return home for washing)
- A list of their preferences (See information for staff in the event of a hospital admission on the next page)

Yourself:

- *Finding the light in dementia* – you can write down any questions and information from hospital staff in the question sheets

- A pen and paper
- Any legal paperwork that might impact on their care such as power of attorney and a living will
- Moist handwipes to help keep you refreshed
- Phone numbers of family and friends

INFORMATION FOR STAFF IN THE EVENT OF A HOSPITAL ADMISSION

- How your partner likes to be addressed, i.e. their name or title.
- If they have difficulties with communication and what usually helps, e.g. _____ finds it easier to understand when given one or two pieces of information at a time.
  - *Do they wear glasses, a hearing aid?*
  - *How they tend to express themselves.*

- What are their food and drink preferences and if they have any struggles with eating, such as swallowing or chewing, e.g. _____can manage to eat his food with a spoon if cut up into small pieces and likes apple juice.
- Any other conditions they may have been diagnosed or pain they may experience, e.g._____ tends to have pain in her left hip in the night.
- Day to day routine with washing, dressing and going to the toilet, e.g._____ can wash himself if given a flannel and I mime the instructions.

- What their mobility is like, e.g. _____tends to shuffle when walking or needs a stick to steady himself.
- A list of medication and dosages and information on how it is taken, i.e. if your partner has swallowing difficulties, it may be in syrup form, or if they have had a bad reaction to a drug in the past, e.g. I put _____'s pain killer patch on their lower back at 6pm, to help them settle for bedtime.
- Their sleep patterns, e.g. when _____ wakes at night they usually need the toilet, a little snack and a hug.
- Any cultural needs, e.g. food, prayer, the language they now speak, e.g._____ seems to speak more in her mother tongue of Spanish now.
- What usually helps to relax your partner. If they tend to pace or become stressed, e.g. _____ feels comfort when he listens to his playlist on his headphones or _____likes to have her blanket and her wool to fiddle with.
- If they have any specific care and welfare requirements refer to power of attorney, living will, advanced care directive paperwork.
- Their lifestory that includes details of close family and friends, hobbies, interests, job/occupation, where they are from.

Acknowledgements

When I first sat down to write a column for a local newsletter and national newspaper, I didn't foresee the impact that it would have on their readers. I wrote every month about different aspects of how dementia can affect people and considered ways that would help them, based on my knowledge and experience listening to people affected by the condition. I gained much positive feedback and gradually as the months went by I thought of putting them together into a book and here it is. I would like to thank Jo Caulfield from the Mumbles Times and Jane and Andrew Silk from the Mature Times for taking a chance on an unknown writer. I would like to thank all the people whose stories have contributed to this book over time and I wish them all well. Thank you also to John Killick, Suzy Webster and Lorraine Morgan for their wise words when reading through this book at different stages before its publication.

Thank you to the wonderful Martha Bullen, who has imparted her extensive knowledge of the publishing world and has guided me every step of the way, helping me make this happen and for Carole Fawcett's wonderful specialist editing, humour, patience and guidance throughout the process. Thank you also to the phenomenal Jerry and

Michelle Dorris for their creativity and design skills, I could never have wished for a better design and help in laying out the book to make it accessible for all. My gratitude also goes to Jack Canfield and Steve Harrison for their inspiration and expertise and to Dave Holland for his suggestions. I would like to thank Dr. Ann Williams for her generosity and proofreading skills, Dr. Diane Sedgley for her continuing support and encouragement and Professor Cathy Treadaway for her inspiration.

My great thanks go to the miraculous Keith Jones for helping me regain my health and stay well throughout this time and to the indefatigable Angharad Brown for her support throughout the DUETcare years. I would like to thank Karen Davies from Purple Shoots for giving me the ability to make this happen, Professor Mark Goode for helping me believe in myself and to Professors Antony Bayer and Roy Jones from the Cardiff and Bath Memory Teams for imparting their knowledge to me whilst working with them.

Thank you, thank you, thank you, to my wonderful husband Jonathan and sons, Ben and Oliver for their dearest love and much humour to keep me going throughout and my Mum, Rita Holbrook for imparting her stories from her time as a nursing home manager. Finally, I want to express my gratitude to my friends Mari Evans and Theresa McNally, two wonderful nurses for their professional feedback and great friendships, and to Dr. Vicky Richards, Jo Bryant, Jo Berry, Jen Best and Bridget Hennessey who have all supported me throughout the ups and downs of life while writing this book!!

About the Author

D r. Jane M. Mullins is a dementia nurse consultant who has devoted over 25 years to the study and practice of dementia care. Through listening to and supporting people and their families during their diagnosis in memory clinics, caring for them in hospital and in care homes, she has helped throughout all of the stages of their condition. This has also included supporting their partners, families and friends.

Her particular passions are finding ways to communicate through music, nature and art as a way to helping people feel well and valued while living with dementia.

Jane has uncovered certain common features that may help caregivers and the people they care for find better ways of coping. Her extensive practice experience is backed up by expert knowledge gained from attending conferences, lecturing and keeping up to date with research, as well as studying for her Ph.D.: A suitcase full of memories; a sensory ethnography of dementia, where she has explored sensory, creative and intuitive ways of communicating with those living with the condition.

Helping others through your experience

If you have found that *Finding the Light* has helped you and your loved one, please consider sharing this with others by writing a review on Amazon.

Thank you!

Some of the proceeds from
Finding the Light in Dementia, a Guide for Families, Friends and Caregivers
go to dementia related charities and programmes

Made in the USA
Middletown, DE
25 June 2021

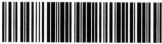